OXFORD MEDICAL PUBLICATIONS

Selected chapters from the Oxford Handbook of Rheumatology

Published and forthcoming Oxford Handbooks

Oxford Handbook of Clinical Medicine 6/e (also available for PDAs and in a Mini Edition)
Oxford Handbook of Clinical Specialties 7/e
Oxford Handbook of Acute Medicine 2/e
Oxford Handbook of Anaesthesia 2/e
Oxford Handbook of Applied Dental Sciences
Oxford Handbook of Cardiology
Oxford Handbook of Clinical and Laboratory Investigation 2/e
Oxford Handbook of Clinical Diagnosis
Oxford Handbook of Clinical Haematology 2/e
Oxford Handbook of Clinical Immunology and Allergy 2/e
Oxford Handbook of Clinical Surgery 2/e
Oxford Handbook of Critical Care 2/e
Oxford Handbook of Dental Patient Care 2/e
Oxford Handbook of Dialysis 2/e
Oxford Handbook of Emergency Medicine 3/e
Oxford Handbook of Endocrinology and Diabetes
Oxford Handbook of ENT and Head and Neck Surgery
Oxford Handbook for the Foundation Programme
Oxford Handbook of Gastroenterology and Hepatology
Oxford Handbook of General Practice 2/e
Oxford Handbook of Genitourinary Medicine, HIV and AIDS
Oxford Handbook of Geriatric Medicine
Oxford Handbook of Medical Sciences
Oxford Handbook of Obstetrics and Gynaecology
Oxford Handbook of Oncology
Oxford Handbook of Ophthalmology
Oxford Handbook of Palliative Care
Oxford Handbook of Practical Drug Therapy
Oxford Handbook of Psychiatry
Oxford Handbook of Public Health Practice 2/e
Oxford Handbook of Rehabilitation Medicine
Oxford Handbook of Respiratory Medicine
Oxford Handbook of Rheumatology 2/e
Oxford Handbook of Tropical Medicine 2/e
Oxford Handbook of Urology

Selected chapters from the Oxford Handbook of Rheumatology

Second Edition

Alan J. Hakim

Consultant Physician and Rheumatologist,
Whipps Cross University Hospital,
London, UK

and

Honorary Consultant Rheumatologist,
University College London Hospital,
London, UK

Gavin P.R. Clunie

Consultant Rheumatologist,
The Ipswich Hospital NHS Trust,
Ipswich, Suffolk, UK

Inam Haq

Senior Lecturer in Medical Education and Rheumatology,
Brighton and Sussex Medical School,
Mayfield House,
University of Brighton,
Falmer, Essex, UK

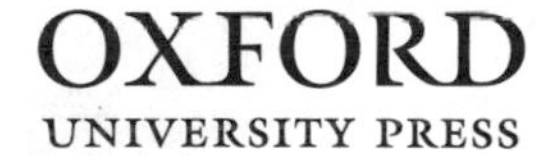

OXFORD
UNIVERSITY PRESS

Great Clarendon Street, Oxford OX2 6DP

Oxford University Press is a department of the University of Oxford.
It furthers the University's objective of excellence in research, scholarship, and education by publishing worldwide in

Oxford New York

Auckland Cape Town Dar es Salaam Hong Kong Karachi
Kuala Lumpur Madrid Melbourne Mexico City Nairobi
New Delhi Shanghai Taipei Toronto

With offices in

Argentina Austria Brazil Chile Czech Republic France Greece
Guatemala Hungary Italy Japan Poland Portugal Singapore
South Korea Switzerland Thailand Turkey Ukraine Vietnam

Oxford is a registered trade mark of Oxford University Press
in the UK and in certain other countries

Published in the United States
by Oxford University Press Inc., New York

First published 2002
Reprinted 2003
Second edition printed 2006
Merck Sharp and Dohme edition printed 2008

British Library Cataloguing in Publication Data
Data available

Library of Congress Cataloging in Publication Data
Hakim, Alan.
Oxford handbook of rheumatology / Alan J. Hakim, Gavin P.R. Clunie.
p. ; cm.—(Oxford medical publications)
Includes bibliographical references and index.
1. Rheumatology—Handbooks, manuals, etc. I. Clunie, Gavin P. R. II. Title.
III. Title: Handbook of rheumatology. IV. Series.
[DNLM: 1. Rheumatic Diseases—Handbooks. WE 39 H155o 2006]
RC927.O952 2006
616.7'23–dc22 2006009451

Typeset by Newgen Imaging Systems (P) Ltd., Chennai, India
Printed in Italy
on acid-free paper by L.E.G.O. S.p.A.

ISBN 978–0–19–956500–9

10 9 8 7 6 5 4 3 2 1

Foreword

Rheumatic or musculoskeletal disorders can present in a number of familiar ways but sometimes are atypical and occasionally bewildering. They may appear insidiously or acutely and their impact ranges from a temporary nuisance, to a condition that is persistent and increasingly disabling, and sometimes a severe, even life-threatening illness.

Not only are they common, and increasingly so in an ageing population, they are often compounded by other disorders associated with ageing. But they affect people of all ages and especially those of working age in whom they are a major cause of sickness absence and curtailment of normal working life. Most do not call for specialist rheumatological care provided the General Practitioner and General Practitioner with a Special Interest are practiced in their diagnosis and treatment, and long-term care. Specialist referral is sought when the diagnosis is uncertain, the treatment ineffective, or a patient is acutely ill, which in some instances will lead to tertiarly referral.

This small book is up-to-date, based soundly on evidence and good clinical practice. It provides a compact but remarkably comprehensive vade mecum both for clinicians in training and trained clinicians who encounter patients with rheumatologic conditions in any guise, and specialists too. Notably, this new edition includes an important chapter on emergencies in rheumatology.

It is a book that I should have been glad to have by me from the beginning of my own career in rheumatology, and I commend it to clinicians today.

Carol Black
Professor Dame Carol Black, President,
Royal College of Physicians, and Professor of Rheumatology,
Royal Free & University College Medical School,
London.

Preface

Rheumatic conditions are common both in general and hospital practice. Musculoskeletal symptoms are a primary feature of many multisystem illnesses, not only in the autoimmune joint and connective tissue diseases, but also metabolic, endocrine, neoplastic, and infectious conditions. Symptoms are also common in the context of injury, age-related change, and psychological distress. Many conditions in rheumatology are a major source of morbidity and mortality.

We have kept to the format of the first edition of this book, focusing first on history and physical signs in the differential diagnosis of rheumatic disease. The reader is then encouraged to consider diseases in more detail. There have been major advances in rheumatology, not least the introduction of biologic therapy. The second edition reflects this in being up-to-date with assessment, guidelines, and treatment options in 2006. We have also introduced several new chapters in Part 2 including one on rheumatological emergencies.

Part 1 offers a practical guide to arriving at an appropriate differential diagnosis given the realistic presentation of rheumatic disease; for example, how to assess someone complaining of a pain in the elbow, knee pain, or of difficulty moving the shoulder, etc. The book suggests appropriate lines of enquiry for patients who present with characteristic patterns of abnormality such as widespread joint or muscle pain, or joint pains in association with a rash. The aim is to provide a guide for obtaining diagnostic information but also for discriminating good from bad information—where to lay emphasis in eliciting a history and examination signs. In most chapters in Part 1, text is laid out under the headings of Taking a history, Examination, and Investigations, with the subheadings indicating important considerations and areas of enquiry.

Part 2 lists a number of rheumatic conditions encountered in rheumatology and general practice. There is a focus on clinical features, specific findings of relevant investigations, and management. There is reference to childhood and adolescent rheumatic disease throughout. The aim is to provide a comprehensive, clinically orientated text. Some reference is made to disease epidemiology and pathophysiology. However, for more detail on the basic sciences the reader is referred to *The Oxford Textbook of Rheumatology*.

Acknowledgements

We would like to thank the editors of *The Oxford Textbook of Rheumatology* third edition and Dr Richard Watts, Dr Mark Lillicrap, and Dr Rachel Jeffery who reviewed the second edition, and the staff at Oxford University Press for their support and encouragement during the preparation of this book.

Contents

Editorial Advisers

Professor David A. Isenberg,
Bloomsbury Rheumatology Unit,
University College London, UK

Professor Peter J. Maddison,
Department of Rheumatology,
Ysbyty Gwynedd, Bangor, North Wales, UK

Professor Patricia Woo,
Centre of Paediatric and Adolescent Rheumatology,
Windeyer Institute,
London, UK

Professor David Glass,
Division of Rheumatology,
Childrens' Hospital Medical Center,
Cincinnati, Ohio, USA

Symbols and abbreviations

⚠	alert/warning
1°	primary
2°	secondary
↑	increase/raise
↓	decrease/reduce
♂	male(s)
♀	female(s)
±	plus or minus
α	alpha
β	beta
AC(J)	Acromioclavicular (joint)
ADM	Abductor digiti minimi
ALP	Alkaline phosphatase
ALT	Alanine transaminase
ANA	Anti-nuclear antibody
ANCA	Antineutrophil cytoplasmic antibody
AP	Anteroposterior
APB	Abductor pollicis brevis
APL	Abductor pollicis longus
APS	Antiphospholipid (antibody) syndrome
AS	Ankylosing spondylitis
ASOT	Antistreptolysin O titre
AZA	Azathioprine
BCP	Basic calcium phosphate (crystals)
BJHS	Benign joint hypermobility syndrome
C	Cervical (e.g. C6 is the sixth cervical vertebra)
CA	Coracoacromial
CINCA	Chronic, infantile, neurological, cutaneous, and articular syndrome
CK	Creatine phosphokinase
CMC(J)	Carpometacarpal (joint)
CPPD	Calcium pyrophosphate deposition (arthritis)
CRP	C reactive protein
CT	Computed tomography
CTS	Carpal tunnel syndrome
CXR	Chest radiograph
dcSScl	Diffuse cutaneous systemic sclerosis

DIP(J)	Distal interphalangeal (joint)
DISH	Diffuse idiopathic skeletal hyperostosis
DM	Dermatomyositis
DVT	Deep vein thrombosis
EBV	Epstein–Barr virus
ECG (EKG)	Electrocardiograph
ECRB	Extensor carpi radialis brevis
ECRL	Extensor carpi radialis longus
ECU	Extensor carpi ulnaris
ED	Extensor digitorum
EDL	Extensor digitorum longus
EDM	Extensor digiti minimi
EHL	Extensor hallucis longus
EI	Extensor indicis
ELMS	Eaton–Lambert myasthenic syndrome
EMG	Electromyography
EPB	Extensor pollicis brevis
EPL	Extensor pollicis longus
ERA	Enthesitis-related arthritis
ESR	Erythrocyte sedimentation rate
FBC (CBC)	Full blood count
FCR	Flexor carpi radialis
FCU	Flexor carpi ulnaris
FDP	Flexor digitorum profundus
FDS	Flexor digitorum superficialis
FHB	Flexor hallucis brevis
FM	Fibromyalgia
FMF	Familial Mediterranean fever
FPL	Flexor pollicis longus
FR	Flexor retinaculum
GCA	Giant cell arteritis
GFR	Glomerular filtration rate
HA	Hydroxyapatite
HIV	Human immunodeficiency virus
HLA	Human leucocyte antigen
HO	Hypertrophic osteoarthropathy
HSP	Henoch–Schönlein purpura
HTLV	Human T-cell leukaemia virus
ILAR	International League ofAssociations for Rheumatology
ITB	Iliotibial band
JCA	Juvenile chronic arthritis
JIA	Juvenile idiopathic arthritis

JIO	Juvenile idiopathic osteoporosis
KD	Kawasaki disease
LCL	Lateral collateral ligament
LDH	Lactate dehydrogenase
LFTS	Liver function tests
lcSScl	Limited cutaneous systemic sclerosis
MCL	Medial collateral ligament
MCTD	Mixed connective tissue disease
MG	Myasthenia gravis
MND	Motor neuron disease
MR	Magnetic resonance
NSAID	Non-steroidal anti-inflammatory drug
OA	Osteoarthritis
OI	Osteogenesis imperfecta
PAN	Polyarteritis nodosa
PCR	Polymerase chain reaction
PIN	Posterior interosseous nerve
PL	Palmaris longus
PLM	Polarized light microscopy
PM	Polymyositis
PMN	Polymorphonuclear neutrophil
PMR	Polymyalgia rheumatica
PSA	Psoriatic arthritis
PSA	Prostatic specific antigen
PTH	Parathyroid hormone
PVNS	Pigmented villonodular synovitis
RA	Rheumatoid arthritis
RF	Rheumatoid factor
RNP	Ribonuclear protein
RP	Raynaud's phenomenon
RS_3PE	Remitting seronegative symmetrical synovitis with pitting oedema
sACE	Serum angiotensin converting enzyme
SAI	Subacromial impingement
SAPHO	Synovitis, acne, palmoplantar pustolosis, hyperostosis, aseptic osteomyelitis (syndrome)
s/c	Subcutaneous(ly)
SLE	Systemic lupus erythematosus
SScl/Scl	Systemic sclerosis/Scleroderma
T	Thoracic (e.g. T5 is the fifth thoracic vertebra)
TB	Tuberculosis
TENS	Transcutaneous electrical nerve stimulation
TFTs	Thyroid function tests

TPMT	Thiopurine S-methyltransferase
TSH	Thyroid stimulating hormone
U&E	Urea and electrolytes
US	Ultrasound
UV	Ultraviolet
WG	Wegener's granulomatosis

Part I

The presentation of rheumatic disease

Chapter 1

Evaluating musculoskeletal pain

Introduction

Pain is the most common musculoskeletal symptom. It is defined by its subjective description, which may vary depending on its physical/biological cause, the patient's understanding of it, its impact on function, and the emotional and behavioural response it invokes. Pain is also often 'coloured' by cultural, linguistic, and religious differences. Therefore pain is not merely an unpleasant sensation; it is in effect an 'emotional change'. The experience is different for every individual.

In children and adolescents the evaluation of pain is sometimes complicated further by the interacting influences of the experience of pain within the family, school, and peer group.

Localization of pain and main pa[illegible]

[illegible]

Localization of pain and pain patterns

- Adults usually accurately localize joint or muscle pain, although there are some situations worth noting in rheumatic disease where pain can be poorly localized (see Table 1.1).
- Pain may be well localized but caused by a distant lesion, e.g. interscapular pain caused by postural/mechanical problems in the cervical spine.
- Pain caused by neurological abnormalities, ischaemic pain, and pain referred from viscera is less easy for the patient to visualize or express and the history may be given with varied interpretations.
- Bone pain is generally constant despite movement or change in posture—in comparison with muscular, synovial, ligament, or tendon pain—and often disturbs sleep. Fracture, tumour, and metabolic bone disease are all possible causes. Such constant, local, sleep-disturbing pain should always be considered sinister and investigated.
- Patterns of pain distribution are associated with certain musculoskeletal conditions, e.g. shoulder girdle muscle pain in polymyalgia rheumatica (PMR) and symmetrical/peripheral joint pain in rheumatoid arthritis (RA). The patterns describe a typical case but are not invariable.
- Patterns of pain distribution may overlap, especially in the elderly where common diseases coexist, e.g. hip and/or knee osteoarthritis (OA), peripheral vascular disease, degenerative lumbar spine.

The quality of pain

Some individuals find it hard to describe pain or use descriptors of severity. A description of the quality of pain can often help to discriminate the cause. Certain pain descriptors are associated with non-organic pain syndromes (see Table 1.2):

- Burning pain, hyperpathia, and allodynia suggest a neurological cause.
- A change in the description of pain in a patient with a long-standing condition is worth noting as it may denote the presence of a second condition, e.g. a fracture or septic arthritis in a patient with established RA.

Repeated, embellished, or elaborate description may suggest non-organic pain, but be aware that such a presentation may be cultural for example.

Table 1.1 Clinical pointers in conditions where pain is poorly localized

Diagnosis	Clinical pointer
Periarticular shoulder pain	Referred to deltoid insertion
Carpal tunnel syndrome	Nocturnal parasthesiae and/or pain, often diffuse
Trochanteric bursitis	Nocturnal pain lying on affected side
Hip Synovitis	Groin/outer thigh pain radiating to the knee

Table 1.2 Terms from the McGill pain scale that help distinguish between organic and non-organic pain syndromes

Organic	Non-organic
Pounding	Flickering
Jumping	Shooting
Pricking	Lancinating
Sharp	Lacerating
Pinching	Crushing
Hot	Searing
Tender	Splitting
Nagging	Torturing
Spreading	Piercing
Annoying	Unbearable
Tiring	Exhausting
Fearful	Terrifying
Tight	Tearing

Eliciting changes in pain by the use of examination techniques

Eliciting changes in pain by the use of different examination techniques may be used to provide clues to the diagnosis:

- Palpation and specific resisted and passive movements can be used to reproduce pain, localizing pathology. For validity, however, a good knowledge of anatomy and a practiced technique are required.
- Given the context in which the examination is done and the effects of suggestibility, manoeuvres should always be interpreted carefully and many experienced clinicians would agree that in certain clinical settings there continues to be a high degree of interobserver variation in diagnosis. Diagnostic examination criteria continue to develop, and many are now validated for research purposes.
- Palpation and passive movement of structures are performed whilst the patient is static. The concept of 'passive' movement is the assumption that muscles and tendons around the joint are removed as potential sources of pain, i.e. one is left just eliciting limitation of movement at the articular surface. This assumption has its own limitations, not least because passive movements of the joint will still cause movement of the soft tissues. In some cases, e.g. shoulder rotator cuff disease, the joint may be painful to move passively because of subluxation or impingement 2° to a musculotendinous lesion.
- The clinician should be aware of myofascial pain when palpating musculotendinous structures, especially around the neck and shoulder regions. Myofascial pain is said to occur when there is activation of a trigger point that elicits pain in a zone stereotypical for the individual muscle. It is often aching in nature.
- Trigger points are associated with palpable tender bands. It is not clear whether trigger points are the same as the tender points characteristic of fibromyalgia.
- Local anaesthetic infiltration at the site of a painful structure is sometimes used to help localize pathology, e.g. injection under the acromion followed by a repeat of an 'impingement test' gauging change from a previously positive test. However, the technique is only reliable if precise localization of injected anaesthetic can be guaranteed. Few, if any, rigorously controlled trials have shown it to give specific results for any condition.

The assessment of pain in young children

The assessment of pain in young children is often difficult:

- Young children often localize pain poorly. Careful identification of the painful area is necessary through observation and palpation.
- A child may not admit to pain but will withdraw the limb or appear anxious when the painful area is examined.
- Observing a child's facial expression during an examination is very important, as is the parent's response.
- Quantification of pain often requires non-verbal clues such as the child's behaviour. Pain rating scales are often helpful (see Fig. 1.1).

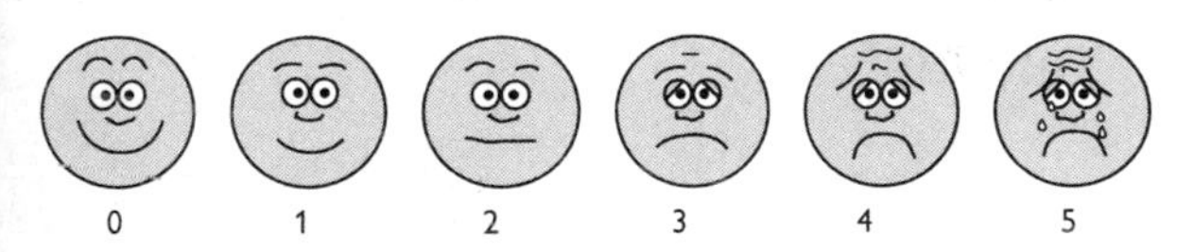

Fig. 1.1 Pain assessment in children—the faces rating scale.

Chapter 2

Regional musculoskeletal conditions: making a working diagnosis

Introduction

This chapter aims to provide a guide to constructing an appropriate differential diagnosis in the patient who presents with regional musculoskeletal symptoms. It does not make reference to all possible diagnoses, only the most common. The section is divided into discussion of the neck, upper limb (shoulder, elbow, wrist), hand, thoracolumbar spine, lower limb (pelvis, groin, thigh, knee), and foot.

General consideratons

- Findings from conventional clinical examination and imaging of the musculoskeletal system usually reflect a static situation. Examination in the context of function (i.e. carrying, lifting, walking, bending, etc.) is not easy, though it is arguably more appropriate. Therefore a thorough history utilizing a good depth of knowledge of functional anatomy is the best alternative and an invaluable way of obtaining good information about abnormal function and its causes.
- Time spent obtaining a detailed account of the onset of symptoms is often helpful whether or not the symptoms are of recent onset or chronic or obviously associated with trauma. Patients usually have a clearer concept of injury-induced disease and may try to rationalize the appearance of non-trauma-related symptoms by association with an event or injury.
- Weakness (as a symptom) may be due to a neuropathic or myopathic condition or it may be perceived according to the impact of other symptoms such as pain.
- With children it is important to obtain a history from both the carer (parent, nanny, or other adult) and the child. Second-hand information, even if provided by the mother, may be less reliable than direct information from the carer.
- Regional musculoskeletal lesions may be a presenting feature of a systemic disorder such as an autoimmune rheumatic disease, malignancy or infection. Clinical suspicion should trigger a common 'screen' of investigations.
- Screening for disseminated malignancy, lymphoma, myeloma, and infection should at least include an FBC, immunoglobulins, ESR, CRP and bone biochemistry. Thereafter tests should be directed specifically towards the clinical scenario.

Corticosteroid injections and rehabilitation, as part of regional pain treatment, are discussed in general terms at appropriate points in the text. The practical approach to these therapies is presented at the end of this chapter.

Neck pain

Background epidemiology

- About 10% of the adult population has neck pain at any one time, although many people do not seek medical help.
- About 1% of adult patients with neck pain develop neurological deficit, but overall levels of disability are lower than for patients with low back pain.
- Isolated neck pain in children and adolescents is unusual. More commonly it accompanies thoracic spine pain or pathology.
- A continuum of radiological appearances exists in relation to age: intervertebral disc narrowing, marginal end-plate osteophytes, and facet joint changes. The appearances are often termed 'degenerative'; however, their correlation with the presence and severity of pain is poor.

Table 2.1 lists the major causes of neck pain in adults.

Functional anatomy

- The neck is the most mobile (37 separate articulations) but least stable part of the spine. There are seven vertebrae (C1–C7) and five intervertebral discs (C2/3–C6/7). The C7/T1 disc is most often associated with radicular symptoms and 'degenerative' disease is common between C5 and T1. If it occurs, cord compression is most likely in this region, though atlantoaxial subluxation may produce the same picture.
- Minor congenital abnormalities are not infrequent and increase the risk of degenerative changes.
- Nerve roots C2 and C3 cover sensation over the back of the head, the lower jaw line, and the neck.
- Nerve roots (C4–T1) leave the spine in dural root sleeves, traverse the intervertebral foramina and form the brachial plexus.
- Cervical nerves have a dermatomal representation (Fig. 2.1) and supply upper limb musculature in a predictable way.

Taking a history

The site, radiation, and description of pain

- Nerve root (radicular) pain is usually sharp and reasonably well-localized in the arms. It is often 'burning' and associated with parasthesiae and numbness. Nerve root irritation and compression by an intervertebral disc are common causes of radicular pain. However, in older adults and those who suffer recurrent bouts of pain it is usually due to encroachment of vertebral end-plate or facet joint osteophytes, or thickened soft tissue/fibrosis on the nerve leading to stenosis of the exit foramen.

Table 2.1 The major causes of neck pain in adults

Soft tissue lesions (posture, psychogenic issues, and overuse as modifiers)	Neck strain
	Torticollis
	Myofascial pain
	Trauma (e.g. acute flexion—extension injury ('whiplash'))
	Cervicothoracic interspinous bursitis
Degenerative and mechanical lesions	Spondylosis
	Disc prolapse
	Thoracic outlet syndrome
	Diffuse idiopathic skeletal hyperostosis (DISH)
Inflammatory conditions	Rheumatoid arthritis (RA)
	Spondylarthropathy (associated with fracture and inflammatory discitis)
	Juvenile idiopathic arthritis
	Polymyalgia rheumatica (PMR)
	Myelitis
Bone lesions	Traumatic fracture
	Osteomyelitis (e.g. TB)
	Osteoporosis (fragility fracture)
	Osteomalacia (bone disease or muscle pain)
	Paget's disease
Non-osseous infections	General systemic infection (general/cervical myalgia)
	Meningitis
	Discitis
Malignancy	Primary (rare) or 2° tumours (and pathological fracture)
	Myeloma, lymphoma, leukaemias
Brachial plexus lesions	Trauma
	Thoracic outlet syndromes (e.g. cervical rib)
Referred pain from	Acromioclavicular or temporomandibular joint
	Heart and major arteries (e.g. angina, thoracic aorta dissection)
	Pharynx (e.g. infection, tumour)
	Lung and diaphragm (e.g. Pancoast tumour, subphrenic abscess)
	Abdomen (e.g. gallbladder, stomach, oesophageal, or pancreatic disease)
	Shoulder (e.g. adhesive capsulitis) (Chapter ?)

- Pain from deep cervical structures is common. It often localizes poorly across the upper back. It can be referred to the upper arms, is typically described as 'heavy' or 'aching' and is more diffuse than nerve root pain.
- Muscle spasm often accompanies various lesions. It can be very painful.
- Pain from the upper cervical spine (C1–C3) can be referred to the temperomandibular joint (TMJ) or retro-orbital regions. Conversely, pain from both TMJ disorders and as a result of dental malocclusion can be referred to the neck.
- Pain from the lower neck may be referred to the interscapula and anterior thoracic wall regions. The latter may mimic cardiac ischaemic pain.
- Florid descriptions of the pain and of its extent and severity are associated with prominent psychological modulators of pain.
- Evaluation of the shoulder joint is often necessary as pathology there often coexists and symptoms around the shoulder often complicate neck evaluation.
- Occipital headache is a common manifestation.

Acute neck pain with trauma

⚠ Acute neck pain with trauma requires urgent assessment even if there are no obvious neurological symptoms:

- Acute trauma requires urgent evaluation and consideration of fracture, spinal cord damage, and vertebral instability. About 80% of serious injuries occur from an accelerating head hitting a stationary object.
- An abrupt flexion injury may fracture the odontoid (this occurs less commonly with extension); however, < one in five injuries at C1/C2 produce neurological deficit because of the wide canal at this level.
- If not traumatic or osteoporotic (the latter being relatively rare in the cervical spine), fractures may occur in bone invaded by malignancy.

New and/or associated symptoms

Ask about associated leg weakness and new bladder or bowel symptoms. New onset acute neck pain with neurological features needs urgent evaluation. Neurological symptoms may also accompany chronic neck pain:

- Spinal osteomyelitis, meningitis, discitis (infection or inflammation), myelitis and fracture may all present with acute or subacute neck pain. All may cause cord compression. Myelopathy due to spondylosis typically presents with a slowly progressive disability over weeks/months, although it can be acute, particularly if associated with central disc prolapse.
- Subacute pain, flaccid paralysis and profound distal neurological signs may suggest myelitis, a condition caused mainly by infections and autoimmune diseases.
- Tinnitus, gait disturbance, blurring of vision and diplopia associated with neck pain are all ascribed to irritation of the cervical sympathetic nerves.

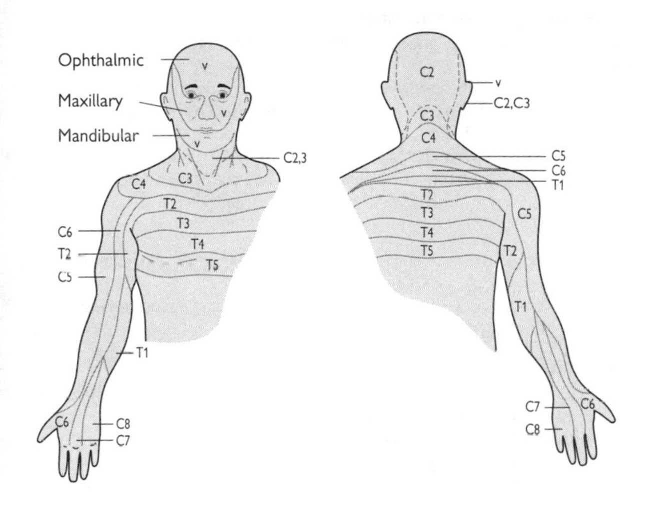

Fig. 2.1 Dermatomal distribution of the cervical and upper thoracic nerves reflecting the radicular pattern of nerve root lesions.

- The vertebral arteries pass close to the facet joints just anterior to emerging nerve roots. Dogma invokes disruption of vertebral blood flow as a cause of dizziness in severe cases of neck spondylosis.

Previous trauma

Ask about previous trauma—it often precedes and influences chronic pain:

- Acute and occupational (chronic overuse) trauma is a common antecedent of chronic neck pain.
- Unresolved litigation associated with trauma is a recognized correlate of the persistence of neck pain and reported disability.
- Cervical dystonia (torticollis) can occur 1 to 4 days after acute trauma, it responds poorly to treatment and can be long-standing. It may also complicate arthropathy such as in RA or Parkinson's disease.
- Whiplash injury is associated with chronic myofascial pain.
- In some patients with chronic pain following, sometimes trivial, trauma there may be dissatisfaction with the quality of care received at the time of the injury.

Occupational and leisure activities

Some occupations and sports/activities are associated with recurrent neck pain:

- Neck pain (and early spondylosis) is prevalent in people whose occupations require persistent awkward head and neck postures, e.g. professional dancers.
- Though biomechanical factors may be an important influence in initiating and aggravating neck pain, there may also be an underlying genetic predisposition to OA and/or hypermobility.

Other points

Establish whether the pain started or varies with any non-musculoskeletal symptoms:

- Cardiac ischaemia, dyspepsia, or abdominal pain can result in referred pain to the neck (see Table 2.9).

Examination

The neck is part of the functional upper limb and symptoms in the arms and legs may be relevant. Neurological examination of the arms is important.

- Inspection from front and back may reveal specific muscle wasting or spasm and poor posture.
- Observing active movements reveals little if the patient has severe pain or muscle spasm. Inability to move the neck even small distances is characteristic in advanced ankylosing spondylitis (AS).
- Tenderness often localizes poorly in degenerative disease. Exquisite tenderness raises the possibility of a disc lesion, osteomyelitis, or malignancy (the latter two are rare).
- There may be 'trigger points' in neck stabilizer and extensor muscles. Activation of a trigger point elicits myofascial pain in a zone that is stereotypical for the individual muscle.
- Tender points (localized, non-radiating pain elicited on thumb pad pressure), notably at the occipital origin of the trapezius, the medial scapular border and the mid-belly of the trapezius, are features of fibromyalgia (FM). It is not clear whether tender and trigger points are the same.
- Examination of passive mobility may be helpful primarily if it reveals gross asymmetry. The normal range of movement varies depending on age, sex, and ethnicity. Generally, at least 45° of lateral flexion and 70° of rotation should be achieved in a middle-aged adult. Global loss of passive mobility is non-specific and occurs with increasing age. The range of movement that might indicate hypermobility has not been established.
- Care should be taken if neck instability is a possibility (e.g. fracture, RA). Vigorous passive examination of forward flexion may exacerbate disc lesions.
- Examination of the shoulder is important to evaluate any referred pain or associated articular lesion (e.g. adhesive capsulitis).
- Neurological examination of upper and lower limbs is important in all cases where pain is referred to the arms and/or the legs if cord compression is a possibility: look for ↑ tone, clonus, pyramidal weakness and extensor plantar response. Check for a cervicothoracic sensory level.

Investigations

Radiographs

Radiographs should be requested with specific objectives in mind:

- A lateral neck film may demonstrate soft tissue thickening in infection or synovium in RA, will document spondylitis (syndesmophytes, discitis and periosteal apposition (in posterior elements associated with psoriasis)), and the severity of spondylosis.
- Oblique views centred on the suspected level may show nerve root foramen stenosis from bony encroachment in patients with radiculopathy. There may be underlying OA.
- High cervical flexion and extension views and a 'through-the-mouth' view are useful to demonstrate odontoid pathology.
- In a patient with RA, if the distance between the anterior arch of the atlas and odontoid process is > 3 mm on a lateral film taken in flexion, there is likely to be C1/C2 AP subluxation.
- On a lateral film superior odontoid subluxation in RA can be judged from a reduced distance from the anteroinferior surface of C2 to a line drawn between the hard palate and base of the occiput (McGregor's line). The distance should be >34 mm in men and >29 mm in women. Lateral odontoid subluxation is best demonstrated with magnetic resonance (MR) imaging.
- Stepwise vertebral subluxation throughout the cervical spine demonstrated on a lateral film is characteristic of (advanced) RA.
- There may be only a few but important signs of spinal infection such as a soft tissue mass or isolated loss of joint space.

Magnetic resonance (MR) and computed tomography (CT)

- MR has largely superceded CT, arthrography, and CT-arthrography in assessing cervical spine/nerve, dural, vertebral, disc, and other soft tissue lesions in the neck.
- In many cases the relevance of some MR 'abnormalities' is still being established—patterns of signal abnormality do occur in asymptomatic people. The frequency of these effects increases with age.
- MR is the technique of choice for imaging disc prolapse, myelopathy, myelitis and for excluding infection or tumours. MR is used to help evaluate the need for, and plan, neurosurgical intervention in high cervical instability in RA patients.
- MR may show soft-tissue swelling around the odontoid in CPPD disease but the diagnosis is best made with CT which shows calcification around the odontoid and of adjacent ligaments ('crowned dens syndrome').
- In patients with the combination of unexplained radiographic signs and generalized symptoms MR is an important investigation. Cases of spinal infection such as TB or brucellosis and lymphoma and can be picked up.

Scintigraphy

- Scintigraphy has little role in diagnosing neck lesions.
- Despite improved image quality and tomographic images, on an isotope bone scan the neck remains one of the most poorly imaged regions of the skeleton and it is non-specific.

Treatment

Table 2.2 shows the principles of treating mechanical cervical syndromes and the timing of MR scanning.

- Remember to review the diagnosis if pain is persistent depite treatment and symptoms seem disproportionate to the results or reports of imaging. In our experience inflammatory psoriatic-related neck pains are often mistaken for 'cervical spondylosis'. This may be because the clinician too readily assumes the latter diagnosis and/or radiologists misreport radiographs.

Table 2.2 The principles of treating mechanical neck syndromes and the timing of mr scanning

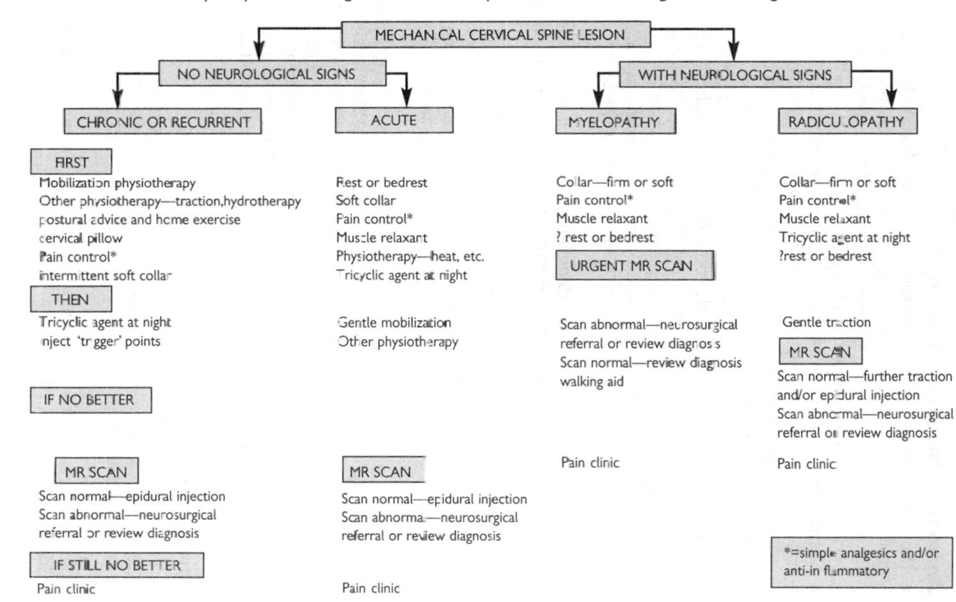

Shoulder pain

Anatomy of the shoulder (see Fig. 2.2)

- The glenohumeral joint is a ball and socket joint. The shallow glenoid cavity permits a wide range of movement. The circular fibrocartilagenous labrum sits on the glenoid and increases the articular surface area and acts as a static joint stabilizer.
- Normal glenohumeral movements include depression then glide and rotation of the humeral head under the coracoacromial (CA) arch to enable elevation of the arm. As the arm elevates there is smooth rotation and elevation of the scapula on the thoracic wall.
- Shoulder movements are a synthesis of four joints: glenohumeral, acromioclavicular (AC), sternoclavicular (SC), and scapulothoracic.
- Movements at AC and SC joints enable slight clavicular rotation, shoulder elevation/depression, and protraction/retraction.
- The rigid CA arch protects the glenohumeral joint from trauma and it, and the overlying deltoid, are separated from the capsule by the subacromial (subdeltoid) bursa.
- A cuff of muscles surrounds the glenohumeral joint capsule. These 'rotator cuff ' muscles are supraspinatus, infraspinatus, teres minor, and subscapularis.
- Supraspinatus initiates abduction by depressing the humeral head then elevating the arm alone for the first 10° of movement. The more powerful deltoid then takes over abduction. Infraspinatus/ teres minor and subscapularis externally and internally rotate the arm in the anatomical position respectively (see Fig. 2.3).
- Production of powerful shoulder movements requires some degree of arm elevation as the larger muscles such as deltoid, latissimus dorsi (extensor), and teres major (adductor) work inefficiently with the arm in the anatomical position. The rotator cuff muscles act synchronously as joint stabilizers throughout the range of shoulder movement.
- The long head of biceps tendon originates above the glenoid usually attached to the labrum and runs within the glenohumeral joint capsule anteromedially in a bony groove.

Pain and shoulder lesions

- Shoulder pain is common and may have its origin in articular or periarticular structures or may be referred from the cervical or thoracic spine, thoracic outlet or subdiaphragmatic structures (Table 2.3).
- Shoulder lesions often produce pain referred to the humeral deltoid insertion (patient points to upper arm).
- Periarticular disorders, mainly subacromial impingement (SAI) disorders, are the commonest cause of shoulder pain in adults (> 90% of cases).

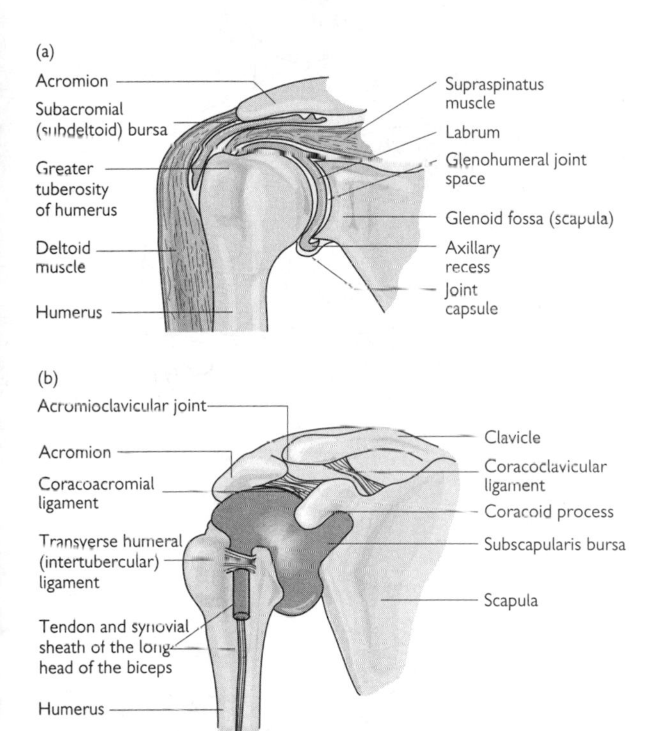

Fig. 2.2 (a) Major shoulder structures. (b) The relationship of the joint capsule to its bony surround and the coracoacromial arch

- Traumatic or inflammatory lesions of many different shoulder structures and conditions that result in neuromuscular weakness of the rotator cuff or scapular stabilizers may result in impingement pain.
- Impingement pain is thought to be generated by the 'squashing' of subacromial structures between the greater tuberosity of the humeral head and the CA arch during rotation/elevation of the humeral head.

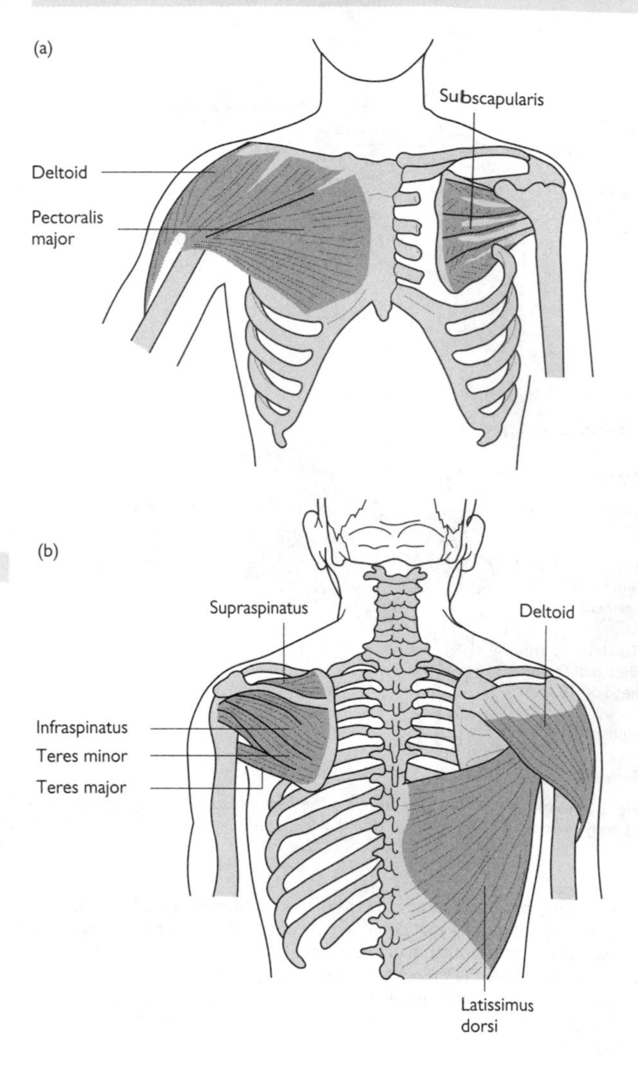

Fig. 2.3 The muscles of the shoulder: (a) anterior view; (b) posterior view

Table 2.3 The commonest causes of shoulder pain

Periarticular lesions (often manifest as subacromial impingement pain)	Rotator cuff tendonitis/tears (very common age 40y+)
	Calcific tendonitis
	Bicipital tendonitis
	Subacromial bursitis
	Milwaukee shoulder (basic calcium phosphate crystal periarthritis)
	Periarticular muscle weakness
Articular lesions	Synovitis (glenohumeral or AC)
	OA (glenohumeral or AC)
	Glenohumeral instability (e.g. labral tears)
	Adhesive capsulitis ('frozen shoulder')
Neurological	Cervical nerve root and radicular referred pain
	Neuralgic amyotrophy
	Spinal cord lesions: tumours, syringomyelia
Neurovascular	Algodystrophy
Thoracic conditions (referred pain)	Mediastinal tumours
	Angina
Systemic and diffuse conditions	Polymyalgia rheumatica
	Myositis
	Chronic pain disorders
	Polyarticular synovitis
Bone disorders	Tumours
	Osteonecrosis
	Paget's disease
Subdiaphragmatic (referred pain)	Gallbladder disease
	Subphrenic abscess

Taking a history

When did the pain start? Injury?

Injurious conditions are common and are both acute and chronic (overuse).

- Rotator cuff lesions (inflammation, degenerative weakness, or tear) are often associated with activities and occupations that involve straining the arm in abduction or forward flexion. A history of an acute 'injury', however, is not always obtained. Subsequent calcification in the tendon following a supraspinatus injury can be asymptomatic or present with acute pain.
- Manual labour (e.g. seamstress) is a risk for rotator cuff lesions. There is typically no acute injury but a history of recurrent provocative movements over years.
- Athletes employed in throwing and racket sports are at risk of rotator cuff tendonopathy and labral tears. Rugby players are at risk of clavicle fracture, shoulder dislocation (and long-term instability), and disruption of the acromioclavicular joint (ACJ).
- Pain from degenerative glenohumeral or ACJ arthritis might be a long-term sequelae of a bone or joint injury.
- The shoulder girdle is one of the commonest sites for a chronic pain syndrome.
- Myofascial pain of the shoulder girdle is common and may mimic the symptoms of cervical radiculopathy and even reflux oesophagitis or ischaemic heart disease.
- Severe, persistent, sleep-disturbing pain of recent onset may be indicative of avascular necrosis, osteomyelitis, or of bony tumours. Though uncommon in the shoulder region these conditions should not be missed.

Where is the pain?

- Pain from the shoulder may be referred to the deltoid insertion.
- Well-localized pain may occur with ACJ arthritis (e.g. patient places a finger on the affected joint) though referred C4 nerve root pain and pain from bone lesions of the distal clavicle is maximal in the same area.
- Glenohumeral articular and capsulitis pain is not well localized (e.g. the patient covers their shoulder with their hand).
- Periscapular pain may be associated with SAI syndromes but may also be myofascial (typically) or referred from the cervicothoracic spine.
- Bilateral shoulder pain should increase suspicion of the presence of an inflammatory polyarthritis such as RA, juvenile idiopathic arthritis, psoriatic arthritis or CPPD arthritis—these would be rare without other joint symptoms.
- Diffuse pain across shoulder girdle muscles in those over 55 years of age raises the possibility of PMR. This pain is often associated with immobility and stiffness.
- A deep aching pain associated with stiffness is characteristic of adhesive capsulitis (frozen shoulder). The use of the term frozen shoulder is popular, though often incorrectly applied. It is a condition that is rare in patients under 40 years of age. The condition is invariably phasic: a painful phase, an adhesive ('frozen') phase, and a resolution

phase. Phases often overlap and the duration varies but long-term limitation of shoulder movement remains in up to 15% of patients. It is associated with diabetes.

Does the pain vary?

Movement- or posture-related pain may be a clue to its cause:

- Rotator cuff lesions often present to rheumatologists with an SAI pattern of pain—that is, pain reproducibly aggravated by specific movements during each day such as reaching up with the arm. Articular, bone, and adhesive capsulitis pain is more likely to be persistent.
- A history of recurrent bouts of shoulder pain in children and adolescents may suggest glenohumeral instability owing to hypermobility or previous trauma, e.g. a labral tear. In an unstable shoulder, pain may result from synovitis, subchondral bone damage, or a 2° SAI disorder. The frequency of recurrent anterior subluxation is inversely proportional to the age at which the initial dislocation occurs.

Are there spinal symptoms?

There is an association between neck conditions and shoulder pain. C4 nerve root pain is referred to the shoulder, adhesive capsulitis is associated with cervical nerve root symptoms (the nature of the link is unknown), and inflammatory neck lesions such as CPPD and psoriatic spondylitis forms can be associated with bilateral shoulder pain referral and can mimic PMR.

Examination

Visual inspection

Inspect the neck, shoulders, and arms from the front, side, and back with the patient standing.

- Abnormality of the contour of the cervicothoracic spine could indicate muscle imbalance/spasm or might be associated with a nerve root origin of pain.
- Scapular asymmetry at rest is especially relevant when examining children and may indicate a congenital bony deformity. Subtle degrees of asymmetry are common and are not usually due to specific pathology nor are they of consequence.
- Diffuse swelling of the whole shoulder may suggest a shoulder effusion/haemarthrosis or subacromial bursitis. In the elderly, possibly Milwaukee shoulder. Swelling of the ACJ occurs with joint diastasis, arthritis and distal clavicular bone lesions.
- Arm swelling and skin changes distally could indicate algodystrophy.

Elicit any tenderness

Eliciting tenderness of discrete shoulder structures is often unrewarding:

- Tenderness of the ACJ, humeral insertion of the supraspinatus tendon, and the long head of biceps tendon may be clues to pathology but palpation will not be specific for diagnosis.
- An appreciation of trigger points associated with myofascial pain and tender points in fibromyalgia is important in the interpretation of regional soft tissue tenderness.

Document bilateral shoulder movements

This aids diagnosis but also gives an indication of the level of functional impairment and can help in monitoring changes over time (Table 2.4). The movements are first tested actively (the patient does the movement) and then passively (the clinician supports the limb). Muscle strength can also be assessed whilst testing active movement.

- Observe arm elevation in the scapular plane from behind, noting symmetry of scapular movement, the pattern of pain during elevation, and the range of elevation. Hunching of the shoulder at the outset of arm elevation often occurs with an impingement problem. A painful arc may suggest a rotator cuff lesion. Inability to lift the arm suggests a rotator cuff tear or weakness, capsulitis, or severe pain, e.g. acute calcific supraspinatus tendonitis.
- Observe and compare internal rotation of shoulders judged by how far up the back the hand can reach. Poor performance may be due to weakness of cuff or scapular stabilizing muscles or pain, usually as a result of subacromial impingement. This manoeuvre assumes normal elbow function.
- Observe the range of external rotation of the humerus from the front. Ask the patient to flex their elbows as if they were holding a tray and rotate the arms outwards. Minor degrees of restriction caused by pain are not specific but severe restriction is characteristic of adhesive capsulitis.

Test for subacromial impingement

- Always compare the affected with the non-symptomatic side and make conservative judgments about muscle weakness if there is pain impeding voluntary effort.
- Most tests rely on their ability to narrow the distance between the humeral head and the CA arch, by driving the greater tuberosity under the CA arch as the humerus rotates (see Fig. 2.4).
- Whether the tests are specific for lesions of the subacromial structures or for the site of impingement is unknown.

Movement of the glenohumeral joint

Move the glenohumeral joint passively in all directions by moving the upper arm with one hand and placing the other over the shoulder to feel for clunks, crepitus, and resistance to movement:

- If the humeral head can be slid anteriorly (often with a 'clunk') clearly without rotation in the glenoid it suggests instability.
- Grossly reduced passive shoulder movement (notably external rotation, with or without pain) is the hallmark of adhesive capsulitis.
- Pull down on both (hanging) arms. If the humeral head moves inferiorly (sulcus sign) there may be glenohumeral instability.

Table 2.4 Isolated muscle testing of shoulder girdle muscles

Muscle: nerve root, peripheral nerve supply and muscle action	Muscle position	Isolated muscle test	Common pathology affecting muscle strength/bulk
Supraspinatus: C5/C6. Suprascapular nerve. Initial humeral abduction and stability of raised upper arm	From behind, seen and felt above the scapular spine at rest and when activated	Abduct arm from neutral against resistance	Tear or disuse following damage, e.g. after a fall, chronic overuse stress, or in athletes (throwing arm)
Infraspinatus: C5/C6. Suprascapular nerve. External rotation and stability of humeral head	From behind, seen and felt arising from medial scapular border passing laterally (below the scapular spine)	External rotation of arm in neutral,elbow supported and flexed at 90°	Tear or disuse following chronic damage
Serratus anterior: C5–C7. Long-thoracic nerve. Pulls the scapula forward on the thoracic wall (extends forward reach of arm)	Appreciated from behind when patient is pushing against a wall with arms outstretched in front, in that scapula remains fixed	Test by pushing wall with an outstretched arm or push-up. If paralysed there will be lifting andlateral excursion of the scapula	Damage to long-thoracic nerve from trauma. Patient may also have SAI
Deltoid: C5/C6. Axillary nerve. Flexion, extension but mainly abduction of humerus	Arises from the scapular spine and acromion, then swathes the shoulder inserting into the humerus laterally	Wasting may be obvious. Weakness in isometric strength of an arm abducted to 90°	Lesions of axillary nerve damaged by anterior shoulder dislocation (external rotation may also be weak from denervation of teres minor)

Stress the acromioclavicular joint

Stressing the ACJ may reproduce the pain. This is conventionally done by compression or shear tests:

- These tests should not normally be painful. Although painful tests have not proved to be specific for ACJ pathology (pain from SAI may also be present), a positive test may provide a clue that the ACJ is arthritic, dynamically unstable, or that impingement of structures in the subacromial space under the ACJ is occurring.
- Hold the patient's arm in forward flexion (90°) and draw it across the top of the patient's chest. The resulting compression of the ACJ may produce pain. ACJ pain can also be elicited by passively elevating the arm through 180° bringing the hand to the ceiling. Pain is experienced in the upper 10° or so of movement.

Shoulder examination with the patient supine

Examine the shoulders with the patient supine to test whether there is anterior cuff deficiency, glenohumeral joint laxity, or a labral tear: this is especially important in young adults and adolescents to identify an 'unstable shoulder'. Hold and support the upper arm held in slight abduction and external rotation (the elbow is flexed). Move the arm gently (cranially in the coronal plane) and apply gradual degrees of external rotation.

- Deficiency of anterior structures is suggested by patient apprehension that pain is imminent or that the shoulder will slip forward. With a labral tear there may be an audible/palpable 'clunk'.
- Pressure downward on the upper arm (taking the pressure off anterior shoulder structures by an anteriorly translocated humeral head) may relieve this apprehension or the pain associated with it (positive relocation test).
- An unstable shoulder identified with the above tests may denote previous traumatic injury (e.g. shoulder dislocation) or a hyper-mobility disorder.

Investigations

The optimum initial imaging for investigating undiagnosed shoulder pain is disputed. Some clinicians advocate management of shoulder problems based on history and examination alone. This is a practical approach to a common problem as, it is said, many problems get better in the short-term. The long-term sequelae of such management strategies, where a firm diagnosis has not been made, are unknown however. Studies of shoulder pain in Primary Care suggest that chronic shoulder problems are common, often despite initial improvement.

(a)

Painful arc
(active)

Action: Patient standing. Slow arm abduction (scapular plane).

Positive test: Pain onset (maximal) at (variable) angular range.

(b)

Neer test
(passive)

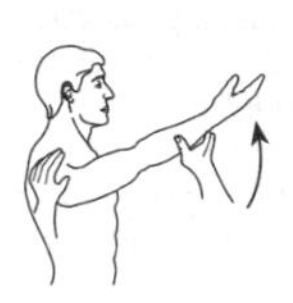

Action: Patient sitting/standing. Passive forward flexion. Scapula fixed.

Positive test: Pain at (variable) angle of flexion.

(c)

Empty can
(active)

Action: Patient sitting/standing. Active forward flexion to 90° then internal rotation—'can empties'.

Positive test: Pain with flexion or rotation of arm.

(d)

Kennedy–Hawkins
(passive)

FIX

Action: Patient sitting/standing. Passive forward flexion (90°). Fix elbow with hand. Passive internal rotation.

Positive test: Pain at some stage of elevation or rotation.

Fig. 2.4 Tests useful for eliciting subacromial impingement

Radiographs

- The standard projection for screening purposes is anteroposterior (AP), though the AP axial–lateral view taken with the arm abducted may add information about the relationship of the glenoid and humeral head. Look for calcific deposits in soft-tissue (possible basic calcium/phosphate crystals: Milwaukee Shoulder).
- Supraspinatus outlet views are often used to assess acromial configuration and identify inferior acromial osteophytes in patients with SAI.
- If recurrent dislocation is suspected, associated humeral head defects may be identified by an AP with internal humeral rotation or a Stryker view. Bilateral films distinguish anomaly (invariably bilateral) from abnormality.
- Bilateral AP ACJ views with the patient holding weights may identify, and grade degrees of, ACJ diastasis. Distal clavicular erosion may be due to RA, hyperparathyroidism, myeloma, metastases, or post-traumatic osteolysis.
- Though characteristic patterns of abnormality are associated with SAI, minor age-related radiographic abnormalities may normally exist.

Other imaging: ultrasound, arthrography, CT arthrography, MR, bone scintigraphy

- Ultrasound scoring systems for locating and grading rotator cuff tears now exist. The technique permits examination of the rotator cuff with the shoulder in different positions but is highly operator dependent.
- Patterns of rotator cuff abnormality and subacromial impingement are well recognized with both arthrography and MR. However, there is no consensus about which of ultrasound, MR, or arthrography is most accurate for detecting rotator cuff tears.
- Children, adolescents, and young adults with suspected unstable shoulders should have an MR examination as detailed views of the humeral head, glenoid labrum, periarticular glenohumeral soft tissues, and subacromial area are important.
- MR is the imaging of choice in young adults where instability is diagnosed. Rotator interval lesions and labral abnormalities are best assessed with MR. Enhancement with IV contrast may increase the chance of detecting a labral tear.
- No specific patterns of bone scan abnormality have been consistently recognized for isolated shoulder lesions, although a three-phase study may be diagnostic for algodystrophy in the upper limb.

Other investigations

- Local anaesthetic injection may help disclose the site of shoulder pain, although it is possible that by the time anaesthesia occurs the injected anaesthetic has spread to areas not intended as a target.
- Joint aspiration is essential if infection is possible. Fluid is usually aspirated easily from a grossly distended shoulder capsule. Haemarthroses can occur in degenerate shoulders (often in association with chondrocalcinosis), haemophilia, trauma, and pigmented villonodular synovitis.

- Electrophysiological tests may confirm muscle weakness and help establish the presence of neuromuscular disease, e.g. myositis or neuralgic amyotrophy.
- Blood tests are required if looking for infection, inflammatory disease, etc.
  - A normal creatine kinase (CK) will rule out myositis in the majority of cases.
  - Blood urea, electrolytes, creatinine, alkaline phosphatase (ALP), calcium, phosphate, thyroid function tests, and myeloma screen should be considered if metabolic bone or myopathic disease is considered.

Treatment

- Physiotherapy should play a focal part in encouraging mobilization of the joint, and early assessment is recommended. The following principles are recommended:
  - know whether there is an additional neck/spinal generated pain component (physiotherapists are independent diagnosticians and many physiotherapists erroneously aim therapy at cervicothoracic segments for individual shoulder lesions).
  - do not refer to physiotherapy without knowledge of who will see the patient.
  - do not refer to physiotherapy without knowing the approach taken by the specific physiotherapist for instability and rotator cuff weakness.
- Simple analgesics are often necessary.
- Local steroid injections can be considered in the following situations:
  - tendonitis of the rotator cuff
  - adhesive capsulitis
  - ACJ pain
  - subacromial bursitis.
- The principles of steroid injection and rehabilitation are dealt with in the last two sections of this chapter.
- There are several situations where local steroids should be avoided:
  - bicipital tendonitis (rest, analgesia, physiotherapy).
  - the first 6 weeks of an acute rotator cuff tear.
  - where symptoms have become chronic and conservative therapy has not helped for a presumptive clinical diagnosis (this requires reassessment, imaging and a diagnosis as surgery may be required).
- Surgical intervention may take the form of subacromial decompression arthroscopy, synovectomy of the SCJ and ACJ, or excision of the distal end of the clavicle.
  - subacromial decompression may be necessary for chronic rotator cuff tendonitis especially where imaging has shown inferior acromial osteophytes.
  - other interventions include repair of a rotator cuff or biceps tendon rupture and joint replacement (for pain relief rather than improvement in function mainly).
- Lithotripsy does not offer advantages over steroid injection and physiotherapy for calcific supraspinatus tendonitis.

Pain around the elbow

Functional anatomy

- The humeroulnar articulation is the prime (hinge) joint at the elbow, though the radius also articulates with the humerus and, to allow forearm and hand supination/pronation, with the ulna at the elbow (see Fig. 2.5).
- Normal extension results in a straight arm although some muscular people lack the last 5–10° of extension and some (especially women) have up to an extra 10° of extension (hyperextension).
- Normal flexion is to 150–160° and forearm supination/pronation range is about 180°.
- Due to obliquity of the trochlea, extension is associated with slight valgus that can be accentuated in women (up to 15°).
- Unilateral acute traumatic or chronic overuse lesions of the elbow are common. Bilateral symptoms may occur in these situations but be suspicious of referred pain from the neck or possibly an inflammatory articular condition involving both elbows.

Pain may also be referred from proximal neurological lesions in the arm, the shoulder or even from distal lesions such as carpal tunnel syndrome (CTS).

Taking a history

Is the pain exclusively located in the elbow or referred from elsewhere?

Establish whether the pain is associated with neck pain and whether it has neurogenic qualities or is associated with parasthesiae or numbness. There may be referral of pain from C6 or C7 nerve roots, shoulder lesions, or even from compression of the median nerve in the wrist.

Is there a history of acute or chronic (overuse) trauma?

- Pain at the lateral epicondyle 1–2 weeks after a weekend of 'home maintenance' might suggest lateral epicondylitis (tennis elbow) following excessive use of a screwdriver, for example.

Other common sites of pain, where characteristic conditions related to overuse are recognized, include medial humeral epicondyle (golfer's elbow) and olecranon bursa (repetitive pressure/friction). Although typically acute in onset, these conditions may develop insidiously.

- Fractures around the elbow and fractures/dislocations in the forearm are common. Dislocation of the radial head alone is rare and is usually associated with concurrent fracture of the ulna (radiographs may not easily identify the fracture). If not associated with fracture (and especially if recurrent) the condition may be associated with generalized hypermobility or shortening of the ulna due to bone dysplasia.
- In children, a strong pull of the forearm or wrist (occurring primarily in pre-school children) can tear the radioulnar ligament surrounding the radial neck (nursemaid's elbow).

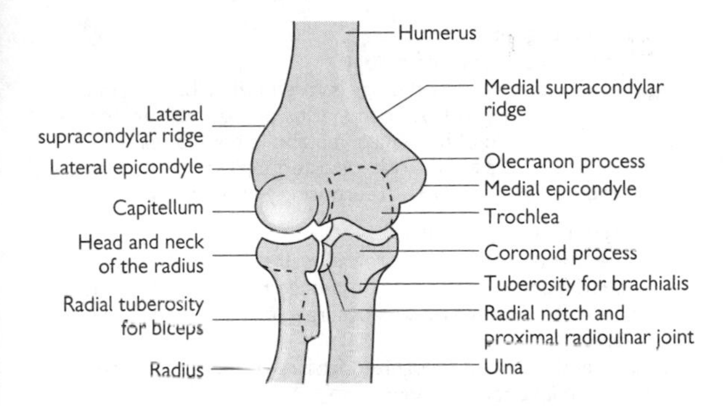

Fig. 2.5 Bony configuration at the (right) elbow (anterior view)

- In children, osteochondritis of the humeral capitellum can occur in mid to late childhood (Panner's disease) typically following repeated trauma.

Does the pain radiate distally?

- Forearm pain may be an additional clue to C6 or C7 radicular pain but may also be due to the spread of musculoskeletal pain along the extensor group of muscles from lateral epicondylitis or rarely from entrapment of the median nerve in the elbow region.
- Associated with occupational overuse, a condition termed peri-tendonitis crepitans is used to characterize symptoms of pain, tenderness, and swelling in the forearm. It is thought to be due to damage of the long wrist/hand flexors and extensors at the muscle–tendon junction.
- Diffuse pain in the forearm can occur as a result of overuse injury, particularly in musicians and typists, though there is overlap with regional pain syndromes.
- Pain around the forearm may also arise from inflammation at the wrist (see the next section) particularly in De Quervain's tenosynovitis.

Is there prominent stiffness with the pain?

- Stiffness is often non-specific but may denote inflammation such as synovitis of the joint or olecranon bursa and, therefore, raises the possibility of an autoimmune rheumatic or crystal deposition disease.
- In the middle aged and elderly, gout of the olecranon bursa and surrounding soft tissues, particularly overlying the border of the ulna, is not uncommon and is often misdiagnosed as infection.

Ask about locking

Locking of the elbow either in flexion or supination/pronation may be due to loose intra-articular bodies. A single loose body is most commonly due to osteochondritis dissecans of the capitellum (e.g. in children with overuse throwing injury – 'Little League elbow') and multiple loose bodies are associated with OA or synovial chondromatosis.

Is the pain unremitting and severe?

This type of pain suggests bony pathology:

- Although non-fracture bone pathology is rare in the elbow region, local bony pain might suggest osteochondritis or avascular necrosis, or, if part of a wider pattern of bony pain, metabolic bone disease.
- In the elderly and others at high risk for osteoporosis, supracondylar and other fractures may occur with surprisingly little trauma.

Are there symptoms in other joints?

Ask about other joints, low back (sacroiliac) pains and risks for gout:

- Elbow synovitis alone is an uncommon though recognized presenting feature of adult RA. Elbow synovitis occurs in children presenting with JIA but is rare (3%).
- Peri-articular enthesitis is a recognized feature of spondylarthropathy (SpA) and may mimic tennis elbow.
- The periarticular tissue around the elbow is a moderately common site for gout.

Examination

Look for abnormality then palpate with the thumb. Observe the active, passive, and resisted active range of joint and related tendon movements and consider examining for local nerve lesions. A complete assessment should include examination of the neck, shoulder, and wrist.

Visual inspection

Look for obvious deformity or asymmetry in the anatomical position:

- Up to 10° of extension from a straight arm is normal. More extension might suggest a hypermobility disorder.
- A child with an elbow lesion typically holds the extended arm close to the body, often in pronation.

Look for swelling or nodules:

- Swelling owing to joint synovitis is difficult to see in the antecubital fossa unless it is florid: it is most easily seen (and more easily felt) adjacent to the triceps tendon insertion.
- The olecranon bursa, which may be inflamed, overlies the olecranon and does not as a rule communicate with the joint. Overlying erythema, although non-specific, may be associated with infection or gout.
- Nodules over the extensor surface or ulna border may be associated with RA.
- Psoriatic plaques are commonly found at the elbow extensor surface.

Observe active flexion and supination/pronation with the elbows held in 90° of flexion:

- Although the range of movement may be affected by extra-articular pain, loss of range usually implies an intra-articular disorder.

Palpate the lateral epicondyle of the humerus

- In lateral epicondylitis (tennis elbow) there is tenderness, which may extend a little distally. Resisted wrist and finger extension with the elbow in extension or passively stretching the tendons (make fist, flex wrist, pronate forearm, then extend elbow) may reproduce the pain.
- Lateral epicondyle tenderness may be due to inflammation of the radiohumeral bursa that lies under the extensor tendon aponeurosis.
- Note that tenderness of lateral and sometimes medial epicondyles can occur in chronic pain syndromes. In these cases, however, the relevant extensor or flexor tendon provocation tests are likely to be negative.

Palpate the medial humeral epicondyle

- Tenderness suggests traumatic medial epicondylitis (golfer's elbow), a regional or chronic pain syndrome, or enthesitis. Confirm the site of the pain by stretching the wrist flexors—supinate the forearm then passively extend both the wrist and elbow simultaneously. Resisted palmar flexion of the wrist or forearm pronation with elbow extension may also cause pain. Tasks that rely on this repetitive movement are often the provoking cause.
- Consider osteochondritis of the medial humeral epicondyle as a cause of persistent pain following an injury. The 8–15-year-old age group is at particular risk as this is a site of 2° ossification.

Passively flex and extend the elbow joint

Passively flex and extend the joint and note the range of movement and 'end-feel' (the feel of resistance at the end of the range of passive joint movement):

- 'End-feel' may tell you whether there is a block to full flexion or extension from a bony spur or osteophyte (solid end-feel) or from soft tissue thickening/fibrosis (springy, often painful).
- Note any crepitus (often associated with intra-articular pathology) and locking (may have loose bodies in the joint).

Supinate and pronate the forearm

Passively supinate and pronate the forearm supporting the elbow in 90° of flexion with your thumb over the radioulnar articulation:

- There may be crepitus or instability/subluxation associated with pain. Instability might suggest a tear or damage to the annular ligament (due to trauma or chronic/aggressive intra-articular inflammation).

Test peripheral nerve function if there are distal arm symptoms

- Given its course around the lateral epicondyle, the integrity of the radial nerve should always be tested when a lateral elbow lesion is suspected.
- The median nerve runs in the antecubital fossa and may be affected in traumatic elbow lesions. It is particularly susceptible where it runs between the two heads of pronator teres (from medial epicondyle and the coronoid process of the ulna) and separates into anterior interosseous and terminal median nerve branches.
- The ulnar nerve lies in the groove behind the medial epicondyle. Bony or soft tissue abnormality in this area may affect nerve function and cause reduced sensation in the little finger and weakness in

(for example) the small muscles of the hand, flexor carpi ulnaris (FCU), extensor carpi ulnaris (ECU), and abductor digiti minimi (ADM). The median and ulnar nerves are dealt with in more detail in the later sections on wrist and hand disorders pp.42–59.

Investigations

Radiographs and other imaging

- Standard AP and lateral radiographs are the most straightforward way of imaging the elbow initially. CT or MR may then be needed if the diagnosis is still obscure and referred pain can be ruled out.
- Look for periosteal lesions and enthesophytes (new bone spurs at clear entheses like the triceps insertion). Periosteal apposition and enthesophytes are typical in psoriatic arthritis.
- A lateral radiograph may identify displacement of the anterior fat pad associated with a joint effusion (sail sign).
- Dislocations of the radial head and associated ulna fractures in children are easily missed. To make this diagnosis a high degree of suspicion and further imaging are often needed.

Needle arthrocentesis/olecranon bursocentesis

- Arthrocentesis/bursocentesis with fluid sent for microscopy and culture should always be done in suspected cases of sepsis. Fluid should be sent for polarized light microscopy in cases of bursitis that may be due to gout. Serum urate is worth requesting but may not be raised even in acute gout.
- Examination of fluid for crystals should always be considered in cases of monoarthritis in the elderly or patients on dialysis.

Electrophysiology

If nerve entrapment is suspected and there is some uncertainty after clinical examination then electrophysiological tests may provide useful information. Testing can help identify the degree and likely site of nerve damage and can help to discriminate between a peripheral and nerve root lesion.

Treatment

- The management of fractures is beyond the scope of this text.
- Epicondylitis is best managed early on with rest, splinting, analgesia, and local steroid injections. The efficacy of physical manipulation has not been proven, though there are theoretical reasons why ultrasound therapy could be of value (it passes through the myofascial planes and concentrates near bone). Resistant cases may benefit from surgery—a 'lateral release'.
- There is anecdotal evidence for the utility of lithotripsy, dry needling, and autologous blood injection for lateral epicondylitis but robust studies showing significant efficacy have not been reported.
- Steroid injections may be of value in the following situations:
  - lateral or medial epicondylitis (hydrocortisone)
  - inflammatory arthritis (usually long acting steroid)
  - olecranon bursitis
  - ulnar nerve entrapment.

The principles of steroid injection and rehabilitation are dealt with at the end of this chapter pp.148–55.

- Surgical procedures include excision of nodules and bursae, transposition of the ulnar nerve, synovectomy, excision of the head of the radius, and arthroplasty.
- Arthroplasty in inflammatory arthritis is best reserved for intractable pain and should be undertaken by an experienced surgeon. Lesser procedures such as proximal radial head excision can be effective to improve pain and function if forearm pronation and supination are poor.
- Radiation synovectomy of the elbow (Y-90 or Re-186) for inflammatory arthritis, PVNS, or synovial chondromatosis requires ultrasound guidance (see EANM guidelines www.eanm.org).

Wrist pain

Functional anatomy of the wrist

- The wrist comprises radiocarpal (scaphoid and lunate) and intercarpal articulations. The ulna does not truly articulate with the lunate but is joined to it, the triquetrum, and the radius (ulnar side of distal aspect), by the triangular fibrocartilage complex.
- The intercarpal joints are joined by intercarpal ligaments and are most stable when the wrist is in full extension. Anterior carpal ligaments are stronger than posterior ones and are reinforced by the flexor retinaculum. Wrist and finger flexor tendons, the radial artery, and the median nerve enter the hand in a tunnel formed by the carpal bones and the flexor retinaculum (carpal tunnel).
- Flexion (70°), extension (70°), radial and ulnar deviation (about 20° and 30° from midline respectively) occur at the wrist but supination/pronation of the wrist and hand is due to radiohumeral movement at the elbow.
- Flexor carpi radialis (FCR) and ulnaris (FCU) are the main flexors of the wrist though palmaris longus (PL) also helps (see Fig. 2.6). All arise from the medial humeral epicondyle.
- All carpal extensors arise from the lateral humeral epicondyle (see Fig. 2.6).
- Radial deviation (abduction) occurs primarily when radial flexors and extensors act together. Ulnar deviation (adduction) occurs primarily when ulnar flexors and extensors act together.

Taking a history

Table 2.5 details the major diagnoses for painful conditions of the wrist and hand.

Determine the exact location of the pain

- Pain localizing only to the wrist is most likely to be from local tissue pathology. Cervical nerve root pain as a result of a C6, C7, or C8 lesion and pain from peripheral nerve lesions is likely to be located chiefly in the hand.
- Pain at the base of the thumb, aggravated by thumb movements, in middle and old age is typical of OA of the trapezium—first metacarpal joint. Pain in this area might also be due to tenosynovitis of thumb tendons.

Trauma history

- Injury/post-injury conditions are common. A history of trauma is important.
- Common fractures in adults are: scaphoid and base of the first metacarpal (Bennett's), and head of the radius (Colles').
- Distal radioulnar physeal injuries may occur in children.
- Post-traumatic chronic wrist pain following injuries may be due to ligamentous injury and chronic carpal instability or osteonecrosis (lunate).

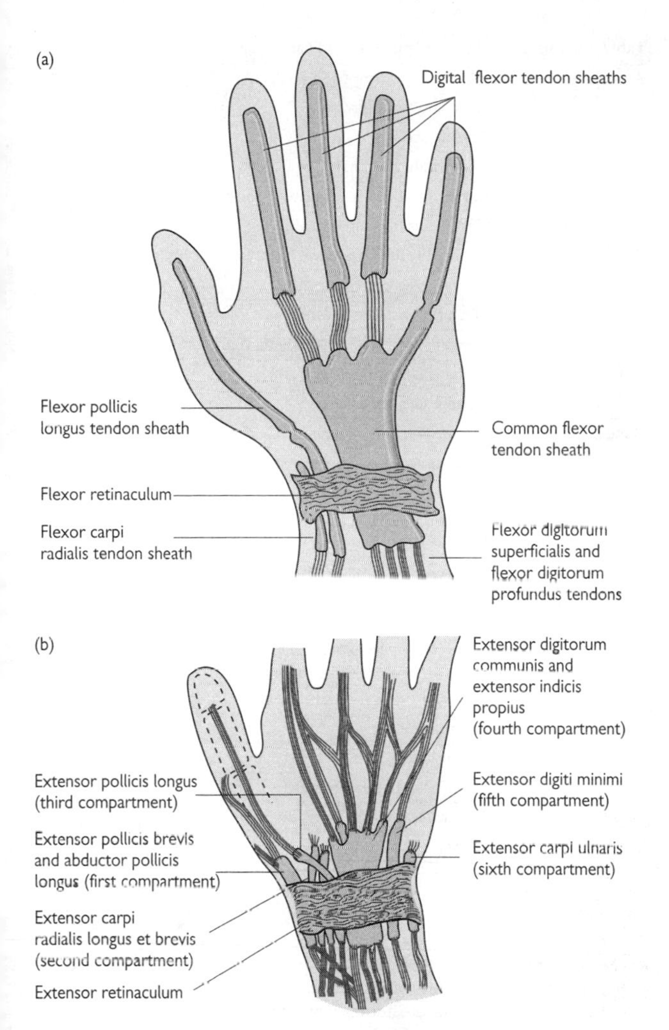

Fig. 2.6 Flexor (a) and extensor (b) tendon sheaths crossing the wrist. Flexor carpi radialis (FCR) inserts into the second and third metacarpals. Flexor carpi ulnaris (FCU) inserts into the pisiform, hamate, and fifth metacarpal. Extensor carpi radialis longus (ECRL) inserts into the base of the second, extensor carpi radialis brevis (ECRB) into the third, and extensor carpi ulnaris (ECU) into the fifth metacarpal respectively

Table 2.5 Painful conditions of the wrist and hand: major diagnoses

Articular disorders	Inflammatory arthritis (e.g. RA, JIA)
	Degenerative arthritis*
	Crystal arthritis
	Ligamentous lesions*
	Carpal instability (e.g. lunate dislocation)
Periarticular disorders	De Quervain's tenosynovitis
	Tenosynovitis of common flexor/extensor tendon sheath
	Flexor pollicis tenosynovitis
	Distal flexor stenosing tenosynovitis (trigger finger or thumb)*
	Ganglia*, subcutaneous nodules, tophi
	Diabetic cheirarthropathy
	Dupuytren's contracture*
Bone pathology	Fracture*
	Neoplasia
	Infection
	Osteochondritis (lunate—Kienböck's; scaphoid—Prieser's)
Neurological	Median nerve entrapment (carpal tunnel* or at pronator teres)
	Anterior interosseous nerve syndrome
	Ulnar nerve entrapment (cubital tunnel or in Guyon's canal in wrist)
	Posterior interosseous nerve entrapment
	Radial nerve palsy
	Brachial plexopathy
	Thoracic outlet syndrome
	Cervical nerve root irritation or entrapment*
	Algodystrophy
	Spinal cord lesions, e.g. syringomyelia

*Common conditions.

- Unusual or florid pain descriptors suggest a regional pain syndrome (e.g. algodystrophy). Following trauma, regional pain syndromes are not uncommon in children, adolescents, or young adults.

Are there features to suggest synovitis?

- Pain due to wrist joint synovitis may be associated with 'stiffness' and be worse at night or in the early morning. Stiffness 'in the hand' may have various causes but these will include multiple tendon/small joint synovitis, diabetic cheirarthropathy, or even scleroderma (Scl).

- Wrist synovitis occurs commonly in adult RA and in children with both systemic and rheumatoid factor positive JIA. It occurs in 5% of oligoarticular JIA cases.
- In the elderly, wrist synovitis may be due to calcium pyrophosphate dihydrate (CPPD) crystals.

The quality of the pain

- Although 1° bone pathology is rare, local bony pain (unremitting, severe, sleep disturbing) might suggest avascular necrosis in those at risk or, if part of a wider pattern of bony pain, metabolic bone disease (e.g. physeal pain in children with rickets).
- Radicular pain may be burning in quality and is typically associated with numbness and parasthesiae. Such neurogenic pain is commonly due to nerve root irritation or compression.

Other joint/musculoskeletal symptoms

- Wrist and extensor tendon sheath synovitis is a common presenting feature of adult RA. Other joints may be affected.
- CPPD arthritis commonly involves the wrist and can mimic RA in its joint distribution and presentation in the elderly.
- Wrist synovitis and enthesitis occurs in SpA. Pain may be considerable though swelling is minimal. There may be inflammatory-type symptoms of spinal pain and enthesitis elsewhere.

Ask specifically about job/leisure activities

- Repetitive lateral and medial wrist movements with thumb adducted can cause tenosynovitis of abductor pollicis longus (APL) or extensor pollicis brevis (EPB) commonly called De Quervain's tenosynovitis.
- If there is no obvious history of trauma, tendonitis may be a presenting feature of a systemic autoimmune rheumatic disease or even gonococcaemia in adolescents and young adults.
- Overuse pain syndromes may occur as a result of repetitive activity. The term 'repetitive strain injury' is controversial. Objective assessment of pain, location of swelling, etc. from the outset is invaluable in assessing the response to treatment. Lack of objective findings (if imaging subsequently normal) suggests a regional pain disorder.

Examination

Visual inspection

Inspect the dorsal surface of both wrists looking for swelling, deformity, or loss of muscle bulk.

- Diffuse swelling may be due to wrist or extensor tendon sheath synovitis.
- A prominent ulna styloid may result from subluxation at the distal radioulnar joint owing to synovitis or radioulnar ligament damage.
- Prominence ('squaring') of the trapezoid–first metacarpal joint commonly occurs in OA of this joint.
- Loss of muscle bulk in the forearm may be 2° to a chronic T1 nerve root lesion or disuse atrophy.

Flexion/extension range tests for major wrist lesions

- The normal range of both flexion and extension in Caucasian adults is about 70° . Synovitis invariably reduces this range.
- Where wrist synovitis is present, swelling on the dorsum of the wrist may become more apparent. Substantial common flexor or extensor tendon swelling will probably also block the full range of wrist movement (soft tissue approximation 'end-feel').
- There is normally an additional 20° of flexion and extension to the active range with passive movement.
- Elicited pain and crepitus are unlikely to be specific for any type of lesion but may draw your attention to the anatomical site of the lesion.

Examine the dorsum of the wrist in detail

- Note any abnormal excursion of the ulnar styloid associated with pain and/or crepitus suggesting synovitis.
- Post-traumatic carpal instability, particularly scapulolunate dissociation, is relatively common. The latter is demonstrated by eliciting dorsal subluxation of the proximal scaphoid pole by firm pressure on its distal pole as the wrist is deviated radially from a starting position with the forearm pronated and the wrist in ulnar deviation. Note any gap between scaphoid and lunate and any associated tenderness.
- Note any tenderness or thickening of the common extensor tendon sheath and tendon sheath of APL and EPB.
- Tenderness at the base of the thumb may be due to wrist synovitis, carpal or carpo–first metacarpal OA, tenosynovitis, a ganglion, or a ligament lesion.
- Finkelstein's test for De Quervain's tenosynovitis may be used to elicit APL/EPB tendon pain. With the thumb adducted and opposed, the fingers are curled to form a fist. Passive ulnar deviation at the wrist stretches the abnormal tendons and elicits pain. Although it is a sensitive test, it is not specific for tendon pain.
- In adults, protrusion of the thumb out of the fist on the ulnar side of the hand during the first part of this test is unusual and suggests thumb, and perhaps general, hypermobility.

Test the integrity of the tendons

Many muscles/tendons that move both the wrist and digits originate at the elbow; therefore, the quality of information gained from isolated tendon resistance tests (either for pain or strength) may be affected by pain elsewhere around the wrist, wrist deformity, or elbow lesions. Interpret findings cautiously. Useful information might be obtained by passive movement of a tendon rather than by resisted active movement, and also by feeling for thickening or crepitus of the tendons.

Investigation and treatment

The investigation and treatment of wrist conditions is covered in the following section on symptoms in the hand.

Symptoms in the hand

Symptoms in the hand are a common presenting feature of some systemic conditions, and localized neurological and musculoskeletal lesions are common, especially in adults. Detailed knowledge of anatomy is beyond the scope of this text. Functional anatomy is important and the more common abnormalities are summarized below.

Functional anatomy of the hand

The long tendons

- Digital power is provided primarily by flexor and extensor muscles arising in the forearm. Their action is supplemented and modified by small muscles in the hand. Precise movements of the hand are mainly due to small muscles.
- Powerful digital flexors (see Fig. 2.6): flexor digitorum superficialis (FDS), flexor digitorum profundus (FDP), and flexor pollicis longus (FPL).
- FDS flexes proximal interphalangeal joints (PIPJs) and, more weakly, metacarpophalangeal joints (MCPJs)/wrist.
- FDP flexes distal interphalangeal joints (DIPJs) and, increasingly weakly, PIPJs, MCPJs/wrist.
- FPL flexes (at 90° to other digits) mainly the PIPJ but also the whole thumb in a power grip (see below).
- Powerful digital extensors (see Fig. 2.6): extensor digitorum (ED) arises from the lateral epicondyle splitting at the wrist to insert into each digital dorsal expansion (digits two to five) that attaches to all three phalanges (see Fig. 2.7). The fifth digit has an additional tendon, extensor digiti minimi (EDM) that also arises at the lateral epicondyle.
- APL abducts the thumb at the MCPJ provided the wrist is stable.
- EPB and EPL extend the thumb.
- Extensor indicis (EI) arises from the ulna posterior border distal to EPL and joins the index finger ED tendon.
- The muscles of the thenar eminence (see Table 2.6) act synchronously. All except adductor pollicis (ulnar nerve, C8/T1) are supplied by the median nerve from C8/T1 nerve roots. All three muscles are supplied by the ulnar nerve (C8/T1).

The intrinsic muscles

- The longitudinal muscles of the palm (four dorsal and four palmar interossei and four lumbricals) all insert into digits.
- Palmar interossei, from metacarpals 1, 2, 4, and 5, insert into dorsal tendons.
- Each dorsal interosseous arises from origins on two adjacent metacarpals. The muscles abduct the second and fourth fingers and move the middle finger either medially or laterally.
- The four lumbricals (see Fig. 2.8, Table 2.7) arise from tendons of FDP in the palm passing to the lateral side of each MCPJ inserting into the dorsal expansions.
- The interossei combine with lumbricals to facilitate fine control of flexion and extension of MCPJs and PIPJs.

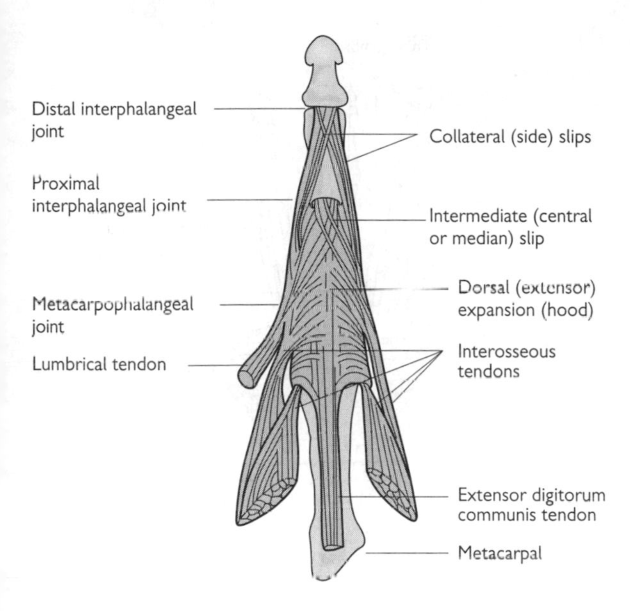

Fig. 2.7 Extensor expansion of a finger

Table 2.6 Muscles of the thenar eminence

Muscle	Origin	Insertion
Abductor pollicis brevis	Flexor retinaculum, scaphoid, and trapezium	Thumb proximal phalanx and dorsal expansion
Flexor pollicis brevis	Flexor retinaculum, trapezium, trapezoid, and capitate	Thumb proximal phalanx (base of radial side)
Opponens pollicis	Flexor retinaculum and tubercle of the trapezium	First metacarpal (lateral border)
Adductor pollicis	Capitate, bases of second/ third metacarpals and distal third metacapal	Thumb proximal phalanx (medial side)

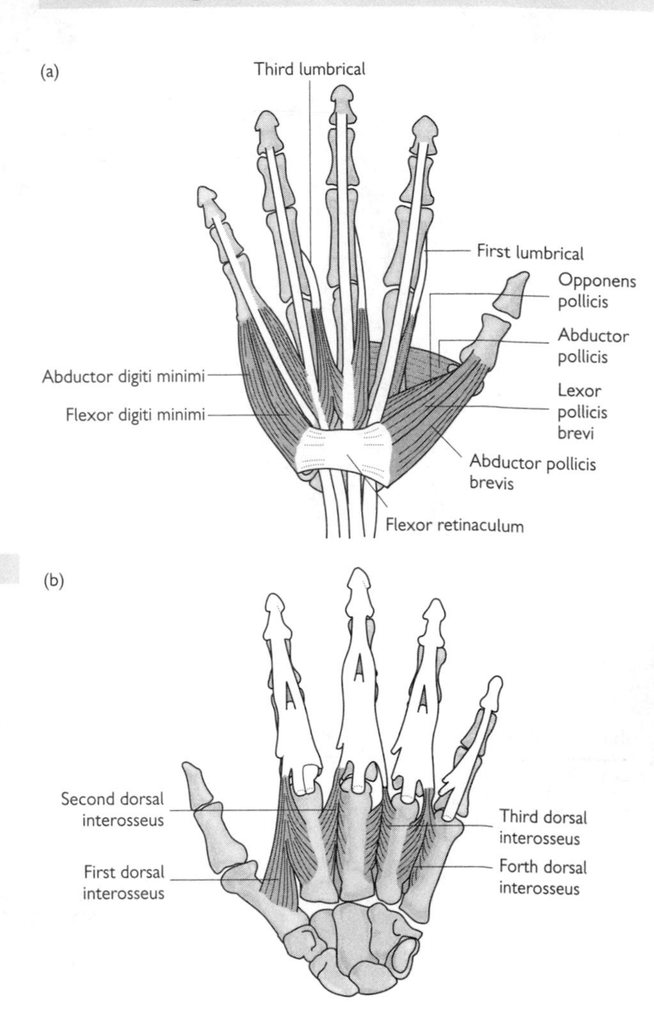

Fig. 2.8 (a) Lumbrical muscles and muscles of the thenar and hypothenar eminences. (b) Dorsal interossei

Table 2.7 Muscles of the hypothenar eminence

Muscle	Origin	Insertion
Abductor digiti minimi	Flexor retinaculum (FR), pisiform, and pisohamate Ligament	Base of the fifth proximal phalanx and dorsal expansion
Flexor digiti minimi brevis	Flexor retinaculum and hook of hamate	Base of the fifth proximal phalanx
Opponens digiti minimi	Flexor retinaculum and hook of hamate	Medial side of the fifth metacarpal

Grip

- For power, the wrist extends and adducts slightly and long digital flexors contract.
- A modified power grip, the hook grip, is used to carry heavy objects like a suitcase. The thumb is extended out of the way and extension at MCPJs accompanies flexion at PIPJs/DIPJs.
- More precision in the grip can be obtained using varying degrees of thumb adduction, abduction, and flexion. The thumb can be opposed with any of the four other digits depending on the shape of the object to be held and the type of manipulation required.

Taking a history

A history of acute or overuse trauma with subsequent localized symptoms requires a straightforward application of anatomical knowledge, precise examination, and judicious choice of imaging techniques for diagnosis. However, there are more subtle or less easily delineated patterns of symptoms in the hand, particularly where pain is diffuse or poorly localized.

Is the pain associated with immobility or stiffness?

- Stiffness may be associated with joint or tendon synovitis but is not specific. Prompting may provide more accurate localization of symptoms.
- If unilateral, especially on the dominant hand, be suspicious that diffuse hand pain may be due to a regional pain syndrome.

Is stiffness local or diffuse?

- Patterns of joint involvement in autoimmune rheumatic disease and polyarticular arthritides are summarized in Chapter 3.
- If localized in the palm there may be Dupuytren's contracture (associated with diabetes). If diffuse, there may be thickening of soft tissue from a systemic process, e.g. hypothyroidism, scleroderma, diabetic cheirarthropathy, or disorders of mucopolysaccharide metabolism (the latter especially in infants, although Fabry's syndrome can present in adulthood associated with acroparasthesiae and palmar telangiectasias).
- Stiffness due to an upper motor neuron lesion (an interpretation of ↑ tone) is unlikely to be confined to the hand and is likely to be associated with weakness. The pattern of symptoms over time should give a clue to its aetiology.

Are there neurological qualities to the pain or characteristics typical of a common nerve lesion?

- 'Burning' or 'deep' episodic pain varying with head, neck, and upper spinal position is typical of cervical nerve root pain. Ask about occupation and other activities that are associated with neck problems, e.g. adolescent ballerina, a seamstress, the relationship with sleep posture, and frequent headaches.
- Pain on the radial side of the hand waking the patient at night and often relieved, at least partially, by shaking the hand is typical of median nerve entrapment in the wrist. However, pain in this condition is often poorly localized at initial presentation. Remember other lesions that produce pain in the area around the thumb base: trapezoid–first metacarpal joint OA, tenosynovitis of APL/EPB (De Quervain's) or EPL, referred pain from a C6 nerve root lesion, and ligament lesions (e.g. ulnar collateral ligament of first MCPJ—'skier's thumb').

Tingling/pins and needles/numbness

Make sure both you and the patient understand what you each mean by these terms.

- Symptoms usually denote cervical nerve root or peripheral nerve irritation/compression though they can reflect underlying ischaemia.
- Tingling in the fingertips of both hands, however, is recognized to occur commonly in patients diagnosed with fibromyalgia.
- Symptoms associated primarily with specific positions of the whole arm may be 2° to thoracic outlet compression of neurovascular structures.

Pain arising from bone

Pain in the hands arising from bones may be difficult to discriminate. Radiographs will often lead to confirmation of the diagnosis.

- The commonest tumour in the hand is an enchondroma. It is usually painless. Once painful then suspect infarction or malignant change.
- Secondary metastases and 1° malignant bone tumours in the hand are rare but must be ruled out in children, adolescents, and young adults with persistent localized bone pain.
- Paget's disease of hand bones can occur but is relatively rare.
- Digital bone pain from osteomalacia/rickets occurs but is unusual at presentation.
- Digital pain may rarely be due to sarcoidosis, hyperparathyroid bone disease, thyroid acropachy, hypertrophic (pulmonary) osteoarthropathy (HO), or pachydermoperiostitis. Look for clubbing.

Ischaemic pain?

A history suggestive of ischaemic pain in the hands is rare in rheumatological practice. Persistent ischaemic digital pain is a medical emergency.

- Digital vasomotor instability (e.g. Raynaud's phenomenon (RP)) is episodic and triggered by cold and emotion, and characterized by digital colour changes: white/blue then red.
- Pain from vasculitis is likely to be persistent and associated with a purpuric rash, nail-fold infarcts, or splinter haemorrhages.
- Ischaemic pain associated with cervicothoracic posture or prolonged arm elevation manoeuvres may be due to a lesion of the thoracic outlet.

- Pain may be due to thromboembolism, e.g. antiphospholipid syndrome, infective endocarditis, or thromboarteritis obliterans (Buerger's disease).

'Swelling'

Examination is more reliable than a history.

- Apart from isolated lesions such as ganglia, patients' description of soft tissue or joint swelling may be unreliable and should be substantiated by examination. Nerve lesions can give the impression that swelling is present (think what a dentist's local anaesthetic does for your lip!).

'Weakness'

Ask about trauma, neck, and median nerve entrapment symptoms.

- Acute tendon injuries are common industrial accidents. Chronic occupational overuse may also lead to rupture.
- If weakness is profound and provided that there has been no obvious trauma, then the cause is likely to be neuromuscular.
- If not associated with pain then weakness is more likely to be neurological than musculoskeletal in origin.
- Weakness associated with pain may be due to a neurological or musculoskeletal lesion, the latter situation often due to an inability to use the hand (or part of it) because of pain or an alteration in biomechanical function as a result of deformity, which may only be slight.
- True weakness associated with stiffness is associated with myelopathy or even motor neuron disease. A detailed history of the progression of symptoms is important and neurological examination should be thorough.

'Catching' of a finger

This may denote stenosing tenosynovitis of a digital flexor tendon (trigger finger). Damage to the tendon and its sheath can result in a fibrous nodule attached to the tendon that moves and catches under the proximal annular ligament just distal to the MCPJ. It may not be painful. This most commonly affects middle and ring fingers and is prevalent amongst professional drivers, cyclists, and those in occupations requiring repeated use of hand-held heavy machinery.

Examination

The sequence below is comprehensive but should be considered if a general condition is suspected. Often an examination only needs to be more specifically directed.

Inspection of the nails and fingers

- Pits/ridges are associated with psoriatic arthritis.
- Splinter haemorrhages may be traumatic but are associated with infective endocarditis or rheumatoid vasculitis.
- Obvious cuticle damage and punctate cuticle erythema (dilated capillary loops) are features of severe RP/Scl.
- Periungual erythema is associated with a number of autoimmune rheumatic and connective tissue diseases.
- Multiple telangiectasias are associated with limited cutaneous Scl (lcScl).

- Diffuse finger thickening (dactylitis) may be due to gross tendon thickening (e.g. SpA or sarcoid), or connective tissue fibrosis/thickening (Scl, cheirarthropathy). Bony or soft-tissue DIPJ or PIPJ swelling should be discriminated.
- A shiny/waxy skin appearance, often pale, may indicate Scl.
- Scattered, tiny, non-blanching dark red punctate lesions are typical of cutaneous skin vasculitis.
- Erythematous or violacious scaly papules/plaques over MCPJs or PIPJs may suggest dermatomyositis.

Note any diffuse swelling of the hand

- Diffuse soft-tissue/skin swelling, may occur in association with RA, RS_3PE syndrome, JIA, algodystrophy, and Scl.
- RS_3PE (remitting seronegative symmetrical synovitis with pitting oedema), which presents mainly in adults in their 70s, may be a distinct type of non-erosive polyarticular/tendon synovitis but may be associated with other, often haematological, conditions.
- Swelling associated with algodystrophy may be localized or diffuse. Skin may be shiny and later there is often a dark red or blue mottled appearance.
- Typical skin appearances are critical to making a clinical diagnosis of Scl. The skin may be initially puffy but later shiny and tight and, with progression, atrophic with contractures.

Note any muscle wasting

Wasting may be due to a degree of chronic denervation (e.g. the thenar eminence in CTS), disuse atrophy (e.g. painful polyarthropathy, joint hypomobility), or ↑ catabolism of muscle (e.g. polymyositis, RA). In the elderly there may be age-related muscle loss.

Note any deformity of digits

- Deformities tend to occur with long-standing polyarticular joint disease, e.g. OA, severe RA, and psoriatic arthritis.
- Isolated deformities may be due to previous bone or tendon trauma, severe neurological lesions and Dupuytren's contracture. A mallet finger (loss of active DIPJ extension) is due to rupture of the distal extensor tendon expansion usually 2° to direct trauma.

Inspect the palm and dorsum of the hand

- Palmar erythema is not specific but is associated with autoimmune disorders of connective tissue and joints.
- Check for Dupuytren's contracture (fascial thickening on ulnar side).
- On the dorsum of the hand, ganglia and swelling of the common extensor tendon sheath are usually easily noted. Swelling of the extensor tendon sheath is commonly associated with RA in adults.

Palpation of joints and nodules

Palpation of joints and nodules is best done using thumb pads with the patient's wrist supported.

- Swelling should be noted for site, consistency, tenderness, and mobility. Osteophytes and exostosis are periarticular or at sites of pressure, may be tender, but are always fixed.

- Ganglia are hard and usually quite mobile (can occur anywhere).
- Rheumatoid nodules (occur anywhere but typically on the dorsum of the hand and the extensor surface of the elbow) and tophi (usually distal) are rubbery, hard, relatively fixed, but may be moved.
- Synovitis is often represented by soft ('boggy'), often springy, swelling around a joint. It may be tender and warm but this is not invariable.
- Synovitis in a single joint may be due to autoimmune rheumatic disease, OA, infection, or foreign-body synovitis (e.g. rose thorn synovitis).

Palpate tendons in the palm or on the volar aspect of the phalanges

- Thickening, tenderness, and crepitus suggest tenosynovitis but tenosynovitis can be hard to spot if it is mild. Tethering and thickening of tendons in the palm associated with excessive digital flexion when the hand is at rest and a block to passive finger extension suggests chronic flexor tenosynovitis (take care to note any contributory joint damage).
- Passive tendon movement by gently flexing/extending a proximal phalanx may disclose palpable tendon nodules, crepitus and tenderness.

Discriminate Dupuytren's contracture from flexor tendonopathy

Dupuytren's contracture typically involves the fourth/fifth fingers (40% bilateral). It is common in males aged 50 to 70. The fascia extends to the second phalanx, thus, if severe, the condition causes fixed flexion of MCPJs/PIPJs. It is associated with epilepsy, diabetes, and alcoholism though is not usually painful.

Investigation of wrist and hand disorders

Radiographs

- An AP view of the hand and wrist is a useful screening investigation to characterize a polyarthropathy and diagnose traumatic and metabolic bone lesions (see Table 2.8).
- Radiographs may reveal soft tissue swelling around joints compatible with a diagnosis of synovitis.
- Radiographs are insensitive for identifying erosions in early autoimmune joint disease.
- An oblique view of the hand may add information about joint erosions if an erosive MCPJ arthritis is considered.
- Lateral and carpal tunnel views of the carpus can be obtained by varying the degree of X-ray projection angle; however, unless searching for evidence of fracture these views are rarely needed.

Further imaging: US, MR, and scintigraphy

- In experienced hands, US patterns of abnormality in association with median nerve entrapment and some soft tissue lesions can be detected.
- In experienced hands, US is a useful way of looking for small hand joint synovitis and erosions in suspected 'early' RA.

Table 2.8 Some conditions/features that may be diagnosed on simple AP hand/wrist radiographs

Bone conditions	Fractures (e.g. scaphoid, base of first metacarpal)
	Tumours
	Metabolic bone diseases (e.g. rickets, hyperparathyroidism)
	Avascular necrosis (e.g. post-traumatic—lunate, sickle cell disease)
	Sarcoidosis (may also have arthropathy)
Specific features	Cartilage damage (joint space loss and subchondral bone changes)
	Articular erosions
	Osteophytes
	Infection (cortex loss, patchy osteolysis)
	Calcium deposition in joint (e.g. triangular ligament chondrocalcinosis)
	Soft tissue swelling (e.g. over ulnar styloid in wrist synovitis)
	Periarticular osteoporosis (associated with joint inflammation)
	Carpal dislocation (e.g. lunate displacement in chronic carpal pain)
Polyarticular/ overall patterns of radiological abnormality	OA (distribution of osteophytes and subchondral bone changes)
	RA, JIA (e.g. deformities, erosion appearance/distribution)
	Psoriatic arthritis (e.g. deformities, erosion appearance—DIPJs)
	CPPD arthritis/gout (e.g. erosion appearance in gout)

- MR may demonstrate a torn or avulsed triangular cartilage in patients with a post-traumatic painful wrist or with carpal instability.
- MR images of the carpal tunnel are especially useful in confirming median nerve compression/tethering and soft tissue wrist pathology, particularly in recurrence of symptoms post-decompression surgery.
- MR can provide valuable information about the degree and distribution of inflammatory disease in joints and tendons, particularly in children and patients where history and examination are difficult.
- MR is more sensitive than radiography in identifying joint erosions in RA. Choosing MR over US depends on availability and sonographer experience.
- Bone scintigraphy is not specific for any single condition but in young adults (after closure of epiphyses and before OA is likely) it may be useful for disclosing patterns of inflammation at and around joints. ^{99m}Tc-labelled human immunoglobulin may be more specific at detecting patterns of synovitis in children and adults.

Laboratory investigations

- FBC, ESR, CRP. The characteristic, though non-specific, picture in patients with a systemic inflammatory condition such as RA or polyarticular JIA, is mild anaemia with normal red cell indices, high or high normal platelets, and ↑ acute phase response. Lymphopenia frequently accompanies autoimmune disease. Neutrophils are raised in infection, with steroids and in systemic JIA or adult Still's disease.
- Blood urea, electrolytes, creatinine, and urate will detect hyperuricaemia and renal impairment associated with gout. Blood calcium, phosphate, albumin, vit D, and ALP (± PTH) will screen for metabolic bone disease.
- Rheumatoid factor (RF) can help characterize but not diagnose an arthropathy (i.e. it is not specific for any one disease). Antinuclear antibody (ANA) and a screen of extractable nuclear antibodies (ENAs) will help characterize any autoimmune connective tissue disease.
- In children with JIA a positive ANA is associated with a risk of uveitis.
- Vasculitis screen, including ANCA in cases of purpuric rash.
- Other investigations to consider: serum angiotensin converting enzyme (sACE) for sarcoidosis, glycosylated haemoglobin in diabetics, serum and urinary protein electrophoresis for myeloma.

Other investigations

- Neurophysiology is a useful adjunct to clinical examination in diagnosis of upper limb neuropathies.
- Joint/bursa fluid aspiration is mandatory in suspected cases of sepsis and should be sent for culture and microscopy. Crystal arthropathy should also be considered.

Treatment of wrist and hand disorders

Treatment for specific diseases is considered in Part 2. Management of the soft tissue lesions in the hand and wrist, like elsewhere, combines periods of rest and splinting with active physiotherapy, avoidance of repetitive activity, and analgesia. In most cases the condition will resolve spontaneously, but severe or persistent pain and disability may warrant input from a hand Occupational Therapist, local steroid injections, or occasionally surgical soft tissue decompression.

- Conditions that respond to local steroid therapy include:
  - tenosynovitis e.g. De Quervain's
  - tendon nodules and ganglia
  - flexor tenosynovitis (and trigger finger)
  - Dupuytren's contracture
  - carpal tunnel syndrome
  - synovitis: radiocarpal and radioulnar at the wrist, MCPJs and PIPJs, first carpometacarpal.
- The accuracy of needle placement is likely to be improved by US guidance; however, greater efficacy from such an approach over blind injection has not yet been shown.
- The principles of steroid injection and rehabilitation are dealt with at the end of this chapter pp.148–53.

- Radiation synovectomy using erbium-169 colloid may be considered useful and, in some cases, may be superior to injecting steroid alone. US guidance of injection of radiocolloid is mandatory.
- Functional evaluation (from a physiotherapist and occupational therapist) is likely to be of use in cases of polyarthropathy. Early use of splints, orthotics, and exercises may lead to greater functional ability and a decrease in symptomology.
- Surgical options for the hand and wrist may include:
  - fusion or resection of the carpal bones
  - ulna styloidectomy and wrist synovectomy (RA)
  - tendon repair and transfer operations (RA)
  - synovectomy of joints and/or tendons (RA)
  - fusion of small joints
  - PIPJ/MCPJ replacements
  - Dupuytren's release/fasciectomy
  - carpal tunnel release
  - trapeziectomy for thumb CMC joint OA

Upper limb peripheral nerve lesions

Background

- Upper limb peripheral nerve lesions are common. Most are entrapment neuropathies. Occasionally, nerve trauma may present to Primary Care physicians or rheumatologists with (primarily) regional muscle weakness.
- Although not specific for its diagnosis, the triad of pain, parasthesiae, and weakness is suggestive of nerve entrapment. Features may be considered more specific for nerve entrapment if there is a history of acute or overuse trauma proximal to the distribution of the symptoms.
- Lesions may characteristically occur in association with specific activities, occupations, or sport (e.g. ulnar neuropathy in cyclists).
- Accurate diagnosis relies on demonstration of the anatomical lesion. Useful in this respect is knowledge of likely sites of entrapment or damage and, in the case of entrapment, the ability to elicit a positive Hoffman–Tinnel sign—percussion over the site of entrapment eliciting sensory symptoms in the appropriate nerve distribution.
- Always compare examination findings in both upper limbs.
- Neurophysiological examination is an adjunct to clinical diagnosis. It should not be relied on to make a diagnosis in the absence of good clinical data.
- MR techniques and their interpretation are becoming increasingly more sophisticated in identifying patterns of abnormality in these disorders.

The long thoracic nerve

- Entrapment is in the differential diagnosis of the cause of painless 'shoulder' weakness. The nerve origin is at C5–C7, and its course runs beneath subscapularis and into serratus anterior.
- Muscle paralysis is often painless and implies loss of the last 30° of overhead arm extension, disrupted scapular rhythm and scapula winging; the latter demonstrated by inspection from behind with the patient pressing against a wall with an outstretched arm.
- Damage to the nerve occurs typically from an anterior direct blow or brachial plexus injury. Damage sometimes occurs after carrying heavy backpacks (e.g. army recruits) or after surgical resection of a cervical rib.
- It can occur spontaneously after infection. There is no specific treatment.

The suprascapular nerve

- The nerve origin is at roots C4–C6, its course is lateral and deep to the trapezius, through the suprascapular notch, terminating in the supraspinatus and posteriorly in the infraspinatus. It carries pain fibres from the glenohumeral joint and ACJ.
- Impingement of the nerve at the suprascapular notch is a cause of shoulder pain where examination and imaging may not reveal an obvious musculoskeletal lesion.
- Injury to the nerve often gives diffuse shoulder pain though painless paralysis of the muscles can occur.

- Injury is often thought to occur from repeated stretching of the nerve at the notch. Weightlifters are prone to bilateral injury and volleyball players prone to dominant side injury.
- Compression by ganglia/tumours occurs and can be confirmed by MR.

Ulnar nerve

The ulnar nerve originates from C8 and T1. It lies along the medial side of the brachial artery in the upper arm, then above the medial humeral epicondyle where it passes posteriorly, piercing the medial intermuscular septum. It then runs behind the elbow in a groove between olecranon and medial epicondyle covered by a fibrous sheath and arcuate ligament (cubital tunnel). Following the line of the ulna in the flexor compartment of the forearm, branches supply flexor digitorum profundus (FDP) and flexor carpi ulnaris (FCU). The nerve enters the hand on the ulnar side dividing into superficial (palmaris brevis and skin over the medial one and a half digits) and deep (small muscles of the hand) branches.

- Lesions are usually due to entrapment.
- The ulnar nerve is occasionally damaged in the relatively exposed cubital tunnel (cubital tunnel syndrome) resulting in pain and parasthesiae along the medial forearm, wrist, and fourth/fifth digits. Damage may occur from direct trauma, compression, or recurrent subluxation. The Hoffman–Tinnel test at the elbow may be positive and there might be sensory loss over the palmar aspect of the fifth digit.
- There are a number of sites where entrapment of the ulnar nerve may occur around the wrist, either proximal to the volar carpal ligament or beneath it or the pisohamate ligament. External compression, acute or recurrent trauma, and ganglia are the usual causes. Symptoms have been noted in cyclists, users of pneumatic or vibrating tools, and in avid videogame players. Entrapment of the purely sensory cutaneous branch can occur from excessive computer mouse use.
- Motor weakness may be most evident by observing general muscle wasting in the hand (hypothenar eminence, interossei, adductor pollicis) and flexion deformity of the fourth and fifth digits—the latter caused by third and fourth lumbrical weakness.
- Flexion of the wrist with ulnar deviation (FCU) and thumb adduction may be weak (adductor pollicis weakness will be evident if you ask the patient to 'run the thumb across the base of the fingers' as normally it can sweep across touching the skin).
- Froment's sign also signifies weakness of adductor pollicis and is demonstrated by a weakness in holding paper between the thumb and the index finger when both are in the sagittal plane.
- Discrimination of a wrist site from an elbow site of nerve entrapment is helped by the site of a positive Hoffman–Tinnel test, preservation of power of wrist flexion/medial deviation (FCU) in a wrist lesion and electrophysiology.
- Rest, analgesia and occasionally local steroids are helpful. A review of posture, repetitive activity, and a biomechanical assessment with changes in activities and technique are recommended. Surgical decompression may also be necessary.

Radial nerve

The nerve origin is at roots C5–C8, and its course runs anterior to subscapularis then passes behind the humerus in a groove that runs between the long and medial heads of triceps. It then winds anteriorly around the humeral shaft to lie between brachialis and brachioradialis. In the flexor compartment of the arm it divides at the level of the lateral epicondyle into superficial branch (cutaneous/sensory) and the posterior interosseous nerve (PIN), which runs through the supinator muscle into the forearm to supply the extensor compartment muscles.

- Entrapment needs to be considered in those cases of shoulder/upper arm trauma where subsequent presentation includes arm/wrist weakness.
- Compression of the radial nerve in the upper arm causes stiffness in the dorsal arm and forearm, weakness of the wrist, and little finger extension. The triceps is usually unaffected as nerve supply to the muscle leaves the radial nerve proximally.
- Transient compression of the nerve at the site of the medial head of triceps has been described in tennis players.
- Compression can occur as the nerve pierces the lateral intermuscular septum just distal to the radial head and also where the PIN pierces the supinator.
- At this lower site, compression is often a consequence of trauma, may be associated with a positive Hoffman–Tinnel test and local tenderness, and the pain may be reproduced by extreme passive forearm pronation combined with wrist flexion. Symptoms may mimic those of lateral epicondylitis. Surgical exploration may be necessary to confirm a diagnosis.

Median nerve

The nerve origin is from C6–T1 nerve roots. Its course from the brachial plexus runs together with the brachial artery in the upper arm (supplying nothing) then enters the forearm between the two heads of pronator teres (from medial humeral epicondyle and coronoid process of the ulna). It runs deep in the forearm dividing into median and anterior interosseous branches. The median branch enters the hand beneath the flexor retinaculum on the radial side of the wrist. All pronator and flexor muscles in the forearm (except FCU and the medial half of FDP) are supplied by the two branches. The median supplies sensory nerves to the radial side of the hand.

- Entrapment syndrome at the wrist is very common.
- In the rare pronator syndrome, trauma, swelling, or masses between the two pronator heads can cause entrapment giving lower arm pain, parasthesiae, and weakness of forearm pronation. There is local tenderness and reproduction of pain from resisted forearm pronation or wrist flexion.
- Pain in CTS is often present at night and relieved by exercising the hand. Daytime symptoms can persist. Pain can be referred up the arm even to the shoulder. Sensory symptoms are confined to the radial three and a half digits.
- Motor inco-ordination (clumsiness) is a common early feature of CTS.

- Symptoms reproduced by a positive Hoffman–Tinnel's sign (percussion over the volar aspect of the wrist) and Phalen's manoeuvre (volar aspect of the wrist rested on the back of a chair and the hand allowed to fall loosely under gravity, held for one minute) indicates nerve compression.
- A severe or chronic lesion is associated with sensory testing abnormality (see Fig. 2.9) and motor weakness of abductor pollicis brevis (APB), opponens pollicis, and first/second lumbricals.
- Nerve conduction studies are indicated if the diagnosis is uncertain, or if the condition is progressive, motor neuron disease is suspected (thenar muscle wasting marked/progressive with minimal sensory symptoms), dual pathology is suspected, surgical decompression is being considered, and in cases of surgical failure. False negative results occur in 10% of cases.
- MR appears to be more sensitive than US for detecting abnormalities involving the median nerve in/around the carpal tunnel.
- Aetiology of CTS is debated but probably multifactorial. The following are associated: Colles' fracture, trauma, carpal OA, diabetes, inflammatory joint/tendon disease (e.g. RA, scleroderma), ganglia, menopause and pregnancy. Also, hypothyroidism, acromegaly, amyloid, and benign tumours.

Treatment of carpal tunnel syndrome

- Night splinting may be curative, especially early in the condition.
- NSAIDs are helpful if there is underlying inflammatory disease.
- Local steroid injections are of value. If partial remission is achieved consider repeating the injection.
- Surgical decompression is indicated when there is failure of conservative therapy, progressive/persistent neurological changes, or muscle atrophy/weakness.
- Failure of surgical release of the carpal tunnel requires further consideration of underlying causes such as a ganglion or other soft tissue lesion. Reconsider also whether there really is a mechanical/local or perhaps a more subtle cause (e.g. mononeuritis or peripheral neuropathy, entrapment at the pronator or nerve root lesion).

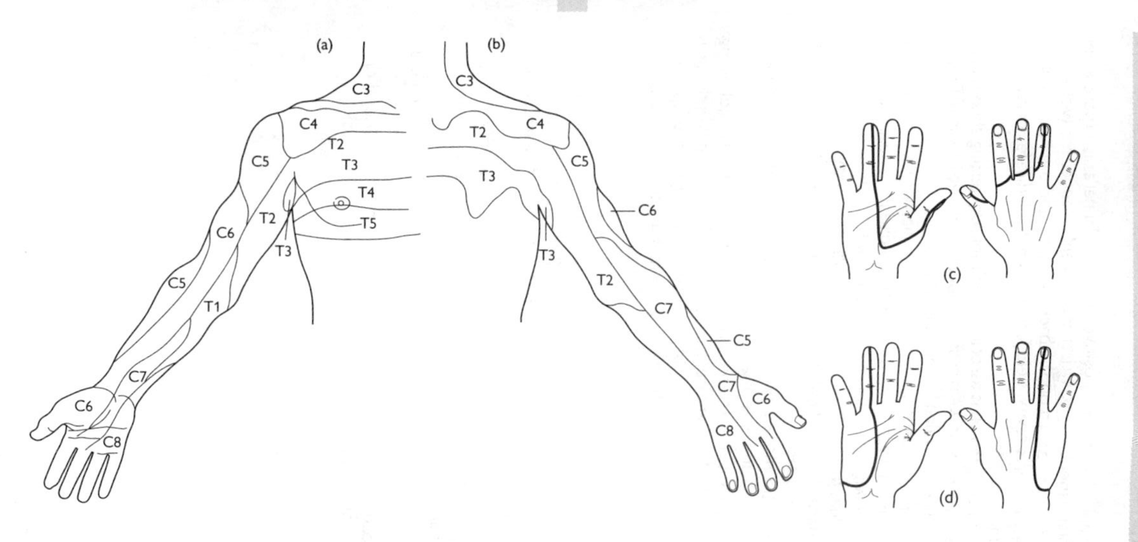

Fig. 2.9 Approximate distribution of dermatomes on the anterior (a) and posterior (b) aspects of the (right) upper limb. Approximate area of sensory change in lesions of the median (c) and ulnar (d) nerves

Thoracic back and chest pain

Background

- The typical thoracic spine (T1–T12) moves less than the lumbar and cervical vertebrae. Segmental movement in any direction is about 6°. However, given the number of segments this can add up to appreciable mobility overall. Less segmental movement results in reduced frequency of problems overall (only 6% of patients attending a spinal clinic have thoracic spine problems).
- Ribs (1–10) articulate posteriorly with vertebrae at two points: the articular facet of the rib head with the costovertebral facet on each vertebral body and the articular facet of the rib tubercle with the costotransverse facet on each vertebral lateral process. These are both synovial joints. Ribs 11 and 12 do not have costotransverse joints.
- The ribs, each continuous with its costal cartilage, articulate anteriorly by synovial joint with manubrium (1–2), sternum (2–7), each costal cartilage above (8–10), or do not articulate (11/12—'floating ribs').
- A massive block of spinal extensor muscles is responsible for maintaining the body against gravity. Some extend over some distance (e.g. the spinalis thoracis from the upper thoracic to the mid-lumbar spinous processes).
- Dermatomes are circumferential and extend from T2 at the clavicles to T10 at the umbilicus. However, up to five nerve roots may contribute innervation of any one point in a truncal dermatome.

Taking a history

The interpretation of cardiac, oesophageal, or pleural chest pain as musculoskeletal in origin is a common occurrence. It may result in missing a serious condition. Take a good history (see Tables 2.9 and 2.10).

- A review of the patterns of quality and radiation of cardiac and oesophageal pain in the clinical context should always be considered.
- Pleuritic pain is common. Recurrent pulmonary emboli are probably underdiagnosed, are difficult to diagnose, and have serious consequences. Any inflammatory, infective, or infiltrative pleural lesion will be painful.
- Lesions confined to pulmonary parenchyma do not produce pain.
- Pericardial pain can be misinterpreted as musculoskeletal or pleuritic.
- Mediastinal abnormalities can produce pain that is often referred.

The interpretation of neurogenic or musculoskeletal chest pains as cardiogenic, oesophageal, or pleural is a common occurrence and may lead to unnecessary investigations. Take a good history (see Table 2.10).

- Thoracic spine lesions can result in referred anterolateral chest pain.
- Costovertebral and costotransverse joint dysfunction is relatively common and is generally age-related but can occur in anyone with spinal deformity. It may produce thoracic spine pain alone or result in an extensive pattern of radiation of pain over the back, lateral, and anterior chest wall.

Table 2.9 Characteristics of chest pain from non-neurological and non-musculoskeletal pathology.

Process	Characteristics of pain
Angina	Gradual onset often related to exercise, a heavy meal, or emotion. Squeezing, strangling, or constriction in chest, can be aching or burning in nature. Commonly substernal but radiates to any of anterior chest, interscapular area, arms (mainly left), shoulders, teeth, and abdomen. Reduces with rest and sublingual nitrates
Myocardial infarction	Similar to above regarding quality and distribution. Longer duration. Less easily relieved
Pericardial inflammation	Sharp or steady substernal pain. Can be referred to shoulder tip, anterior chest, upper abdomen, or back. Often has a pleural component and is altered by change in position—sharper more left-sided when supine but eased by leaning forward
Aortic dissection	Acute onset with extremely severe peak. Felt in centre of chest or back. Lasts for hours
Pleuritic inflammation	Common. Sharp, knife-like, superficial. Aggravated by deep inspiration, sneezing, or coughing. If accompanied by haemoptysis consider pulmonary embolism
Mediastinal conditions	Empyema or surgical emphysema may be intense and sharp and radiate from substernal to shoulder area. Associated with crepitus. Mediastinitis and tumour pain resembles pleural pain. May have constant feeling of constriction/oppression
Peptic disease	Penetrating duodenal ulcers can cause intense, persistent mid-thoracic back pain
Oesophageal reflux	Persistent retrosternal burning is typical. Often post-prandial, when lying or at night/early morning. Oesophageal spasm can be similar to angina and can cause mid-thoracic back pain but reflux symptoms often coexist

Table 2.10 Painful neurological and musculoskeletal conditions of the thoracic spine and chest wall

Thoracic vertebral disease	Osteoporotic or pathological fracture
	Tumours, e.g. osteoid osteoma, metastasis
	Osteomyelitis
	Paget's disease
	Osteomalacia, rickets
	Costovertebral joint dysfunction
Nerve irritation	Root irritation/compression from disc prolapse or osteophyte at exit foramen, from structure distal to exit foramen, or from neuroma
Biomechanical/ degenerative	Scoliosis (non-structural compensatory, structural)
	Diffuse idiopathic skeletal hyperostosis (DISH)
	Calcium pyrophosphate dihydrate disease (of ligamentum flavum)
Herpes-Zoster of intercostal nerve	
Chest wall/superficial lesions	Rib fracture
	Other rib lesions, e.g. tumours, fibrous dysplasia, osteomalacia
	Costochondritis/enthesitis
	Intercostal muscle tear/strain
	Mastitis or fibrocystic disease of the breast
	Myofascial pain and fibromyalgia
	Parietal pleural inflammation/infection/infiltration
Spondylarthropathy (e.g. ankylosing spondylitis)	Spinal inflammation
	Acute discitis
	Chronic indolent discitis
Scheuermann's osteochondritis	In adolescents only

- Lower cervical spine lesions can refer pain to the anterior chest wall.
- Many painful chest conditions are associated with radiation of the pain down the left arm. This pattern is not specific for myocardial ischaemia.
- Lower cervical pain may be referred to the interscapula region.
- Interscapular pain may also be associated with mechanical lumbar disorders. Unlike infection, tumours, and fracture, referred pain is eased or abolished by changes in position or posture.

If there is thoracic back pain alone and it is acute and/or severe consider osteoporosis, tumours, and infection.

- Osteoporotic vertebral collapse is common in post-menopausal women. An acute, non/minimal-trauma-associated severe pain is typical. Fractures occur in many other situations, e.g. AS or a neoplastic bone lesion.
- Spinal infections should not be missed. All are usually associated symptoms. The commonest are *Staphylococcus aureus, Brucella,* and *Mycobacterium tuberculosis.*

Ask about the quality of pain

- Musculoskeletal pain (local or referred) generally associates with specific movements, positions, or postures and is reproducible.
- Pain which increases with coughing, sneezing, or deep inspiration, is suggestive of, but not specific for, pleural lesions. Rib and intercostal lesions or costovertebral joint dysfunction are possibilities.
- Early morning stiffness is not specific for spondylitis and is common. It may be due to muscle spasm associated with a painful lesion.

Ask about other symptoms and risk factors

- The pain from a fracture/lesion (osteoporotic, malignancy, infection) is often localized and extreme, waking the patient at night.
- Acute or chronic thoracic spine lesions may be associated with cord compression. Ask about recent change in sphincter function and progressive lower limb stiffness or heaviness.
- Risks for osteoporosis.
- Systemic symptoms of fever (osteomyelitis).
- Bone pain elsewhere (metastases, osteomalacia, Paget's disease).
- Spinal pain in adolescence (for an adult with kyphosis/spinal pain).
- A positive family history is recognized in idiopathic juvenile scoliosis, osteoporosis, and generalized osteoarthritis.
- Depression and anxiety are important modulators of pain. However, though thoracic back and chest pains may be psychogenic, it is imprudent to settle on this diagnosis without excluding musculoskeletal conditions and diseases of viscera that can cause referred pain.

Examination

Visual inspection

Observe the patient (who has undressed down to their underwear) from back and front. Look for deformity, asymmetry, swellings, and note the respiratory pattern.

- Any scoliosis should be noted. Non-structural scoliosis is frequently due to posture, severe back or abdominal pain, leg length discrepancy, and, rarely, can be psychogenic. Structural scoliosis may be 2° to various lesions at any age.
- There is a normal mild thoracic kyphos; however, marked kyphos in adults (particularly post-menopausal women) might suggest multiple osteoporotic vertebral fractures, though degenerative disc disease often results in kyphosis development in old age. A loss of normal kyphosis (flat spine) may be seen in spondylitis or possibly severe muscle spasm.
- Loose folds of skin on the back might denote multiple vertebral fractures.
- Costochondral swelling occurs in some cases of costochondritis or rickets ('rickety rosary') in children. Look for synovitis of costosternal or sternoclavicular joints (pattern associated with spondylarthropathy).

Palpation

Palpate over the vertebrae, paravertebral joints, and back musculature with the patient prone. Palpate the anterior chest wall.

- Spinal osteomyelitis may be associated with obvious skin swelling and erythema, exquisite focal tenderness, and extensor spasm. Tumours may give similar signs, though skin erythema is not likely.
- Costotransverse joints may be tender (4–5 cm from midline). Discomfort at any costovertebral joint and its referred pain can be elicited by individual rib manipulation (downward pressure on the rib lateral to its vertebral joints when the patient is prone).
- Identify any trigger points that reproduce myofascial pain in back muscles.
- Tender swelling of the sternoclavicular, costomanubrial or sternocostal joints may suggest spondylarthropathy or SAPHO (synovitis, acne, pustulosis (palmoplantar), hyperostosis and (aseptic) osteomyelitis).
- Inflammation of costal cartilages is often associated with painful swelling and tenderness. Rib/intercostal lesions should be easily discriminated from referred pain by eliciting local tenderness.

Check thoracic spinal movement

Movements of the thoracic spine should be checked. Ask the patient to sit on the couch with their arms folded in front of them. Guided by movements of the spinous processes gauge the range of thoracic spine movement.

- Approximate normal ranges of movement in the above position are extension 30° , lateral flexion 30° , flexion 90° , and rotation 60° .
- Scoliosis is often associated with rotation that is accentuated on flexion.

- Abnormal mobility will not be specific for any underlying condition but may draw attention to the major affected spinal segment (painful segments are 'guarded' and may appear hypomobile).
- Spondylitis may become obvious if there is extensive spinal hypomobility.
- Chest expansion should be measured from forced expiration to complete inspiration measuring at expansion, with a tape, at the level of the xiphisternum. Normal young adult chest expansion should measure at least 3 cm.

Other examination

- Given the range of serious conditions causing chest pains, a full medical examination is important and should always be considered.
- Neurological examination of the legs should be considered in anyone who is at risk of spinal cord compression. Look for ↑ tone, pyramidal weakness, ↑ reflexes, and extensor plantars.
- Breast and axillary lymph node examination should be done.

Investigations

Radiographs

- Lateral view radiographs generally provide more information about thoracic spine lesions than anteroposterior views; however, together, both views should confirm osteoporosis, degenerative disease (e.g. previous Scheuermann's osteochondritis, ochronosis, DISH), and Paget's disease.
- Look for vertebral squaring (in AS) and either marginal or non-marginal syndesmophytes as in psoriatic spondylitis or other SpA.
- Discriminate enthesitis from DISH at the corners of vertebrae by the presence of erosions with bone reaction (enthesitis) compared with bone proliferation alone (DISH). Enthesitis, associated with chronic spondylodiscitis is part of the SpA spectrum of diseases.
- Normal radiographs do not exclude malignancy.
- Bone lesions can be well characterized by CT (e.g. osteoid osteoma).

MR

- MR is important in discriminating tumour from infection.
- Disc lesions, spinal canal, and cord are well visualized with MR.
- Fat suppressed or gadolinium-enhanced MR sequences may be necessary to discriminate enthesitis or spondylodiscitis associated with SpA.

Bone scintigraphy

- A bone scan is a sensitive test for infection and malignancy.
- In suspected cases of (previously undiagnosed) malignancy, it is more sensitive than radiographs, can often confirm the lytic or sclerotic nature of a lesion, and will identify any other skeletal sites of disease.
- It is a useful investigation in patients with malignancy who present with back pain. A lack of additional lesions strongly suggests against a single spinal abnormality being malignancy-related.
- Tomography can discriminate abnormality in the pars interarticularis, facet joint, and disc/vertebral body.

- Bone scintigraphy sensitively identifies rib and, in most cases, inflammatory intercostal lesions. If solitary the differential diagnosis is of a metastasis, 1° malignant or benign bone tumour, healed rib fracture, fibrous dysplasia, Paget's bone disease, hyperparathyroidism, or infection.

Other investigations to consider in patients with chest pain

- CXR, then consider pulmonary ventilation/perfusion scintigraphy and spiral CT (?PEs).
- CT of the chest in patients with unexplained pleural pain.
- ECG (EKG) and an exercise ECG or coronary perfusion scintigraphy for patients with possible cardiac ischaemia.
- Transthoracic echocardiography to show thickened pericardium or an effusion associated with pericarditis.
- Upper gastrointestinal endoscopy in suspected cases of peptic ulceration.
- Diagnostic trial of a proton pump inhibitor in cases of reflux oesophagitis.

Treatment

For treatment of thoracic and chest wall lesions see the next section on Low back pain.

Low back pain and disorders in adults

Epidemiology

- The lifetime prevalence of back pain is 58% and the greatest prevalence is between 45 and 64 years of age.
- There are 12 million primary care consultations and over 2.4 million adult outpatient visits to hospitals annually for low back pain in the United Kingdom (population 65 million).
- Estimated annual financial costs of back pain to the United Kingdom National Health Service are more than £500 million. Indirect costs are estimated to be more than £5 billion for lost work.
- The financial health care and indirect employment costs of low back pain in the United States are estimated to be more than $24 billion.

Lumbar and sacral spine anatomy

- There are normally five lumbar vertebrae. Anomalies are not uncommon at the lumbosacral junction.
- The transition between the mobile lumbar spine (flexion, extension, and lateral flexion) and fixed sacrum together with high weight-loading combine to make the region highly prone to damage.
- The facet joints are sharply angled, effectively reducing rotation in lumbar segments.
- The sacroiliac joints (synovial) are held firmly by a strong fibrous capsule and tough ligaments. The amount of normal movement (essentially rotation) is normally inversely proportional to age.
- The spinal cord ends at L1/L2. Nerves then run individually, are normally mobile in the spinal canal, and together are termed the cauda equina.
- Each nerve exits its appropriate lateral intervertebral exit foramen passing initially superior and then laterally to the disc, e.g. L4 from L4/L5 exit foramen. However, in the spinal canal each nerve descends immediately posterior to the more proximal intervertebral disc before it exits. Thus, for example, L4 root symptoms can occur from either lateral herniation of the L4/5 disc or posterior herniation of the L3/L4 disc (or from both).
- Facet joint innervation is from posterior 1° rami, each of which supplies the corresponding joint at its level, one higher and one lower.

Basic principles of assessment

- Low back pain can arise from damage or inflammation of the thoracic or lumbar spines or from the posterior pelvis. Pathology in retroperitoneal abdominal and pelvic viscera can result in referred pain to the low back.
- A simple way of categorizing back pain is to consider its cause to be primarily mechanical or inflammatory, due to bone pathology, as referred pain, or from intrinsic neurological disease (see Table 2.11).
- Over 90% of episodes of low back pain in adults are mechanical, self-limiting, and do not require investigation.

Table 2.11 Common and/or serious causes of low back pain in adults

Mechanical/degenerative (very common)	Hypermobility
	Facet joint arthritis
	Disc disease (annular tear, internal disruption, prolapse)
	Scoliosis/kyphosis
	Spinal stenosis
	Sacroiliitis
Inflammatory (uncommon)	AS
	Sacroiliitis (e.g. AS, brucellosis)
Infection (rare)	Osteomyelitis (e.g. Staphylococcus aureus, TB, brucellosis)
Bone disease (common)	Osteoporotic fracture
	Paget's disease
	Osteomalacia
Neoplasia (rare)	Secondary metastases
	Multiple myeloma
Other	Sickle cell crisis
	Renal disease (e.g. tumours, infection)
	Gynaecological disease
	Fibromyalgia

- Indicators for further investigation include age > 55 years of age, stiffness, focal pain, pain that disturbs sleep, nerve root symptoms, and chronic persistent (> 6 weeks) pain.
- The low back is often a focus for those who may use pain (consciously or unconsciously) as a protective device in the face of domestic, emotional, or occupational stress. These stresses commonly influence the description and impact of pain but rarely act alone in causing pain—there is usually some underlying organic pathology.

Taking a history

Differentiate whether the pain is likely to be primarily mechanical or inflammatory, due to bone pathology or referred

- The site and extent of the pain does not easily discriminate the cause. All disorders may be associated with mechanical deformity and/or muscle spasm that may cause pain in a more diffuse distribution.
- Generally, pain due to mechanical lesions is often acute in onset whereas patients with pain from inflammatory lesions often present after symptoms have been present for some time.

- Inflammatory pain is often worse at night, is associated with stiffness at night/rest or on waking, and is eased by movement. Mechanical lesions often settle at night and worsen with (at least some or certain) movements. Many 'mechanical' or 'degenerative' lesions may have an inflammatory component, e.g. internal disc disruption causing discogenic pain.
- Intrinsic bone pathology often causes severe, unremitting, focal pain. Sleep is disturbed. Pain does not ease substantially with movement.
- About 3% of patients presenting with back pain have non-muscu-loskeletal causes. In the low back (in women) a significant proportion have pelvic conditions such as ovarian cysts or endometriosis. Pain may be cyclical.
- For those aged over 55 with no previous similar episodes of pain—increase suspicion of an underlying neoplastic lesion. Investigation is required.
- Associated systemic symptoms are common in osteomyelitis and may be present if a malignancy has disseminated.

Ask about pain radiation and symptoms in the legs

- Progressive neurological leg symptoms suggest a worsening/expanding lesion such as a tumour, infection/vertebral collapse, Paget's disease, or lumbosacral spinal stenosis.
- Pressure on neural elements of the cauda equina sufficient to cause a disturbance in perineal sensation and/or bowel/bladder paralysis is a neurosurgical emergency (cauda equina syndrome).
- Leg pain caused by nerve root irritation/compression is often clearly defined and sharp, often accompanied by numbness or parasthesiae. The commonest involved nerve roots are L4, L5, or S1. Pain generally radiates to below the knee and often, but not always, to the heel and big toe.
- Sciatic nerve entrapment at the level of the piriformis muscle can produce identical radicular symptoms to L5 or S1 nerve root entrapment.
- Neurological symptoms in the distribution of the femoral nerve (primarily anterior thigh musculature) might suggest a high lumbar nerve root lesion (L1–L3 for example).
- Disc prolapse is the commonest cause of nerve root pain but bony encroachment at the nerve root exit foramen by vertebral end-plate or facet joint osteophytes and/or soft tissue thickening or fibrosis can cause similar pain too (foramenal stenosis).
- Discs do not need to prolapse to cause pain. Annular tears and internal disruption (?microfractures in vertebral end-plates) can cause a pattern of pain, termed discogenic pain, characterized by low back and referred buttock/posterior thigh pain aggravated by movement.
- Generally, all mechanical lesions of the lumbar spine can result in referred pain around the pelvis and anterior thighs. However, pain from lumbar facet joints and probably other segmental structures can be referred to the lower leg.

- Aching in the back and posterior thighs after standing is typical of, but not specific for, spondylolisthesis. There are often added spasms of acute pain, especially if there is segmental instability.
- The symptoms of spinal stenosis are often relieved by sitting bent slightly forward (spinal canal dimensions increase in this position).
- Sacroiliitis often causes referred pain to the buttocks and back of thighs. It occurs commonly in spondylarthropathy.
- Sacroiliac pain can occur in multiparous women—the condition may be associated with hypermobility.

Note the description of the pain

- Pain may be 'severe' whatever the cause; however, note whether the patient's descriptors of it suggest non-organic influences.
- Sharp, lancinating leg pains suggest nerve root irritation/compression (radicular pain) whereas leg pain referred from other structures within a lumbar segment is generally deep and aching. Distribution may be similar (see above). More persistent, rather than episodic, radicular pain may denote stenosis of the nerve root exit foramen.
- A description of bilateral buttock/leg pain that worsens on walking is consistent with spinal stenosis, especially in those with normal peripheral pulses and no bruits.
- A change in the description of pain in someone who has an estab-lished diagnosis may be important, e.g. subacute, severe, unremitting localized pain in a patient with AS who normally has mild inflammatory pain might reflect a superadded discitis; or, acute severe unremitting sleep-disturbing pain in an elderly woman with known chronic mechanical pain associated with OA might suggest osteoporotic fracture.
- Florid descriptions of the pain and its severity are associated with psychological modulators of pain.

Previous back pain and trauma, occupation, and family history

- Scheuermann's disease causes spinal pain in adolescence. It is a risk for spinal degeneration and kyphosis in adults.
- Previous trauma may have caused pars interarticularis fractures (an ante-cedent of spondylolisthesis), vertebral fracture (risk of further mechanical damage), or ligament rupture (subsequent segmental instability).
- It is generally accepted that the high prevalence of disc disease amongst manual workers at a relatively young age provides some evidence for a causal relationship.
- It is often the case that patients with chronic pain following (sometimes trivial) trauma may be dissatisfied with the quality of care received at the time of the injury. Be aware that many believe, and there is some evidence to support this, that the way in which spinal pain is handled at its onset significantly influences its subsequent course.
- Sacroiliitis is an early part of brucellar arthritis (20–51% of patients). Poor animal- or carcass-handling hygiene or ingestion of infected foodstuffs/milk can lead to infection. Spondylitis is a late feature and is characterized by erosions, disc infection, and abcesses.
- A positive family history of low back pain might, in context, suggest SpA (sacroiliitis), hypermobility, or generalized osteoarthritis.

Examination

Inspect the undressed patient from the side and behind

- Note the fluidity of movement when the patient is undressing.
- Check the skin for redness, local swelling, and skin markings. Redness and swelling occasionally accompany osteomyelitis.
- Lipomata, hairy patches, café-au-lait patches, or skin tags often reflect underlying structural nerve or bone abnormality, e.g. spina bifida, diastematomyelia, neurofibromatosis.
- Skin folds often suggest an underlying significant structural change such as osteoporotic fracture or spondylolisthesis.
- Note any deformity: hyperlordosis (associated with L5/S1 damage and weak abdominal musculature), prominent thoracolumbar kyphosis (multiple disc degeneration or vertebral fractures), scoliosis (degenerative, compensatory muscle spasm for unilateral pain).
- Look from the side. A gentle lordotic curve is normal. Flattening suggests muscle spasm or fusion in SpA. With major spondylolisthesis, a step between spinous processes can sometimes be seen.

Observe active movements whilst the patient is standing

Lumbar forward flexion ('...with your legs straight, slowly reach down to try and touch your knees/ankles...'), lateral flexion ('...with your legs and back straight, tip sideways and run your hand down your leg towards your knee...') and extension ('...with your legs straight, slowly bend backwards...'). Note: flexion can be mediated by the hip joints; extension can be effected by slight pelvic tilt and body sway. Ask what can be achieved normally and what is painful.

- Abnormal movements are not specific for any condition though they may help to localize a problem.
- Pain in extension is characteristic of retrospondylolisthesis, facet joint arthritis, or impinging spinous processes. All may be relieved by flexion.
- Failure of the spinous processes to separate in a patient who manages good forward flexion would be consistent with permanent spinal stiffness, e.g. AS, with flexion mediated by the hip joints.
- Forward flexion can be measured using the modified Schöber's test. When erect, mark the skin at the point midway between the posterior superior iliac spines (Venus' dimples) and again 10 cm above and 5 cm below. Measure the increase in distance between the outer marks at full forward flexion—in a young adult this is normally more than 6 cm.
- Ask the patient to stand on one foot then lift onto their toes a few times. Weakness might imply an L5 nerve root entrapment (gastrocnemius/soleus).

Observe the gait pattern

Abnormality of gait may reflect any spinal or lower limb problem:

- An antalgic gait.
- A wide-based gait suggests unsteadiness (due to dizziness, muscular weakness, proprioceptive, or cerebellar deficit etc.).

- Leaning forwards/stiff legged—though not specific, in older people this may denote spinal stenosis.
- Shuffling, which could suggest Parkinsonism (back pain/stiffness is a recognized early sign).
- Foot drop, which could suggest L5 or S1 nerve root compression.
- Flat feet, hind feet valgus, and genu recurvatum on stance phase, might suggest general hypermobility associated with various low back lesions.

Check extension and lumbar rotation (patient seated)

With the patient seated on the couch, check lumbar extension and rotation (the pelvis is now fixed).

- Typically, combined rotation and extension can elicit pain from arthritic facet joints. It is a sensitive though not specific test.
- Slumping forwards (see Fig. 2.10) stretches the dura. Increased lumbar pain may be elicited in cases of disc prolapse but, more importantly, leg pain can be elicited in cases of nerve root entrapment. A more provocative test can be done by gently extending each knee in turn in the slump position. Look for asymmetry.

Examine the sacroiliac joints and hips (patient supine)

With the patient supine, examination of the sacroiliac joints and an examination of the hips should be done to exclude pain arising from these structures.

- Test flexion and the rotational range of each hip by lifting the leg, flexed at the knee, so that the upper leg is vertical. Passive movement should normally be pain-free.
- No SIJ stress test is specific. Tests are designed to reproduce pain in cases of SIJ dysfunction or sacroiliitis. Here are two:
  - press down/out reasonably firmly over both anterior superior iliac spines at the same time.
  - lift one leg, flex, and abduct the hip slightly. Exert an axial force into the acetabulum at two or three different angles. This test is considered by many to be more useful and probably stresses both the joint and many of the sacral ligaments though is less specific if the hip joint is abnormal.

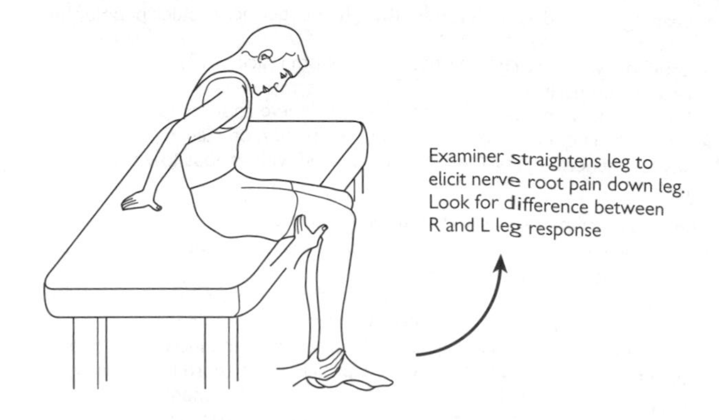

Fig. 2.10 The slump test identifies pain from lumbar disc and nerve root irritation or compression (see text).

Straight leg raise (Laseague's test)

The normal variation in straight leg raise ranges from 60° to more than 90° in adults. Compare sides.

- Discomfort from normal tightening of the posterior thigh or calf muscles must be discriminated from a positive test. A positive test (leg raising restricted to 40° or less by the radicular pain) is most specific in patients aged <30 years and for L5 or S1 nerve root lesions.
- A crossed straight leg raise (pain elicited by raising the unaffected leg) is even more specific for nerve root entrapment.
- To identify more subtle cases of nerve root entrapment, apply additional foot dorsiflexion at the maximum possible angle of (pain-free) leg raise.
- Laseague's test does not always reproduce pain in every patient who has sciatica. It is also often negative in older patients with the condition when it is chiefly due to foramenal stenosis and when central posterior disc prolapse occurs (giving bilateral sciatica but no root compression).

Neurological examination

- Neurological examination of the legs is essential in suspected cases of nerve root entrapment, cord compression, spinal stenosis and cauda equina syndrome.

Table 2.12 lists tests for muscle strength in the lower limbs—weakness may denote nerve root entrapment—and Table 2.13 lists the principal signs of lumbar nerve root lesions.

Table 2.12 Testing muscle strength in the lower limbs (patient supine unless otherwise stated). Weakness may denote nerve root entrapment

Muscle or muscle group	Nerve roots	Test*
Hamstrings (knee flexion)	L5, S1, S2	Ask patient to flex the knee to 45°, hold patient's ankle and ask them to bend the knee further against your hold
Iliopsoas (hip flexion/internal rotation)	L1, L2, L3	Ask patient to lift the leg with a bent knee, hold up the upper leg and resist your push. Try to push the leg down and slightly outwards
Quadriceps femoris (hip flexion, knee extension)	L2, L3, L4	1. Hold the patient's relaxed upper leg above the couch (grasped underneath above the knee). The lower leg should drop loosely. Ask them to straighten the lower leg against your resistance
		2. From patient standing test repetitive squatting for more subtle weakness
Tibialis anterior (ankle dorsiflexion). Tibialis posterior (ankle inversion and dorsiflexion)	L4, L5	1. With the knee straight ask the patient to pull back their foot (show them first) against your pull. Resist dorsiflexion
		2. Standing or walking on heels tests for more subtle weakness. Note: if the hindfoot rests in valgus or the patient significantly everts the foot during dorsiflexion, the test may also recruit peroneal muscles (L5, S1)
Extensor hallucis longus	L5, S1	Ask the patient to pull their big toe back against your finger (at the base)
Gastrocnemius and soleus (ankle plantar flexion)	S1, S2	1. Ask the patient to point their toes. Resist the movement by pressing against the ball of the foot
		2. Standing or walking on the toes tests for more subtle weakness

* Compare sides. Score according to scale, for example: 0 = no muscle contraction; 1 = contraction visible; 2 = active movement, gravity eliminated; 3 = active movement against gravity. 4–/4/4+ = active movement against slight/moderate/strong resistance; 5 = normal power.

Table 2.13 An *aide-mé moire:* principal combinations of signs used for identifying lumbar nerve root lesions

Nerve root	Parasthesiae and sensory change	Muscle weakness	Tendon reflex changes
L2	Upper thigh: anterior, medial + lateral surfaces	Hip flexion and adduction	None
L3	Anterior surface of lower thigh	Hip adduction + knee extension	Knee jerk possibly reduced
L4	Anteromedial surface of lower leg	Knee extension, foot dorsiflexion + inversion	Knee jerk decreased
L5	Anterolateral surface of lower leg + dorsum/medial side of foot/toe 1	Hip extension and abduction. Knee flexion. Foot/toe 1 dorsiflexion	None
S1	Lateral border + sole of foot. Back of heel + calf	Knee flexion. Plantar flexion and *eversion of foot*	Ankle jerk decreased

Examination of the prone patient

Ask the patient to turn to lie prone. Palpate low back and over sacrum.

- Diffuse tenderness may be due to muscle spasm.
- Superficial tenderness over the spinous processes or interspinous interval might suggest interspinous ligament disruption or impinging processes.
- Paravertebral bony tenderness may suggest facet joint arthritis.
- Loin tenderness could indicate renal pathology.
- Tenderness over the SIJs is not specific for sacroiliitis.
- A positive femoral stretch test reproduces L1–L4 (especially L3) radicular pain in the anterior or medial part of the thigh. Flex the patient's knee to 90° and passively extend the hip.

Other examination

- In suspected cases of spinal stenosis or cauda equina syndrome it is essential to check for sensory loss in the sacral nerve dermatomes. Also check anal sphincter tone by rectal examination (S5).
- In suspected cases of spinal stenosis, the patient can be asked to walk until limited by pain then re-examined. If there is any ischaemia of the cauda equina or of a nerve root (from foramenal stenosis) nerve root signs may become more obvious.

Investigations

- There are two important initial steps in investigating low back pain. First deciding whether radiographs will help. Second, though relatively rare in practice, the possibility of infection, malignancy, and cauda equina compression always needs to be borne in mind. Simple radiographic views are insensitive indicators of these conditions and, in most cases, are not specific although most radiologists would agree they are desirable in addition to CT or MR. Laboratory tests are mandatory in all suspected cases of inflammation, infection, and malignancy.

Radiographs—decision-making in requesting them

(Table 2.14)

- Lumbar spine radiographs are not always helpful. Remember that nine out of ten cases of back pain in the primary care setting are mechanical and self-limiting. Features on a plain radiograph of the lumbar spine correlate poorly with the presence or pattern of pain.
- Spondylosis is common, age-related, and often isn't symptomatic.
- Children, athletes, and young adults with back pain need prompt radiographic investigation. Failure to detect and treat a pars interarticularis fracture may lead on to a spondylolysis. Abnormalities are more readily appreciated in these age groups as the frequency of age-related degenerative changes in the spine is low
- Obtaining radiographs to help in the management of patients is a different issue to obtaining them to aid diagnosis and one that requires careful thought, e.g. is the patient likely to perceive that they have received suboptimal care if a radiograph is not requested?

- Spondylolysis may be seen on a lateral view but is more easily seen on oblique views. Oblique views will also show pedicle stress fractures in athletes.
- Spondylolisthesis may be identified and graded by a lateral film. Flexion and extension views may be helpful in delineating subtle cases and instability (spondylolytic).
- General osteopenia is a risk factor for low bone mass; however, it is not a sensitive indicator of low bone mass.
- Look for vertebral squaring (in AS), non-marginal syndesmophytes (other SpA e.g. psoriatic) or the flowing or exuberant syndesmophytes of DISH.
- Consider obtaining an AP view of the pelvis. Established, but often not early, sacroiliitis can be ruled-out. A further 'coned' view is often helpful.
- Sacroiliitis (periarticular osteoporosis, erosion, sclerosis of bone, widening joint space) occurs in all types of SpA. It can be unilateral.
- Sclerosis of the SIJ on the lower iliac side alone suggests osteitis condensans ilii. Joint space is normal and joint margin well defined.
- Patterns of metabolic bone disease, Paget's disease and hip pathology are usually readily identifiable on a pelvic film.

Bone scintigraphy

- A bone scan is an extremely sensitive test for infection or malignancy. It is a useful investigation in patients with previously diagnosed malignancy who present with back pain, especially in those who have had no previous skeletal metastases. A lack of additional lesions strongly suggests against a single spinal abnormality being malignancy-related.
- It is not specific for the various degenerative lesions but can help localize the site of a lesion.
- Bone scan SIJ appearances in sacroiliitis can be unreliable.

CT or MR?

The choice of imaging depends largely on likely clinical and radiographic differential diagnosis:

- For spondylolytic spondylolisthesis, CT shows the exact site of pars' defects. The usual appearance is of sclerotic irregular edges.
- Nerve impingement can be shown by CT or MR.
- Intervertebral disc prolapse, both posterior and posterolateral, can be shown by either technique. Prolapse material is of similar CT density and MR signal to the disc and well-defined against epidural fat.
- Changes in the normal disc signal pattern are associated with age-related disc degeneration. Discogenic pain has been associated with MRI abnormalities classified according to Modic.
- On T_2-weighted MR, disc material is usually of higher signal than 'scar' (e.g. fibrosis from a previous lesion), in which signal decreases with aging. Recent scarring enhances immediately but old scarring does so only slowly. This discrimination requires gadolinium-enhanced MR.
- CT or MR shows early sacroiliitis in AS when X-rays are normal.

Table 2.14 Commonly reported patterns of radiographic abnormality in adults, the interpretation, and suggested reaction.

Radiographic abnormalities	Lesion suggested	Sensible further action
Lumbosacral anomalies	Risk for future back pain	May not be clinically significant. Risk for low back pain (esp. if hypermobile)
Generalized osteopenia	Osteoporosis	Measurement of bone density. Rule out secondary causes, e.g. myeloma
Narrowed disc space, marginal vertebral end-plate osteophytes or both	Intervertebral disc disruption	MR if persistent symptoms or signs of same level nerve root entrapment, spinal or nerve root exit foramen stenosis
Localized lucent or sclerotic lesion, loss of cortex	Tumour, infection, or fracture	Discuss case with radiologist. MR or CT may be advised. A bone scan may be helpful. Initiate appropriate laboratory tests immediately
Facet joint OA	Facet joint syndrome	Consider whether there is associated spinal/nerve root exit foramen stenosis ('radicular symptoms) or symptoms suggestive of spondylolisthesis. CT or MR is then likely to be appropriate
Pars interarticularis defect	Spondylolysis/ ?spondylolytic	Probable prior fracture. Further oblique film centered on suspected level or CT should confirm. Association with symptoms or signs of disc disease or spondylolisthesis suggests an unstable segment. Flexion and extension lateral view radiographs may show instability. MR helpful for imaging soft-tissues including nerves
Short lumbar pedicles	Spinal stenosis	Consider MR if symptoms suggest spinal stenosis
Mixed patchy sclerosis and lucency in entire (enlarged) vertebra(e)	Paget's disease	Neurological leg symptoms suggest spinal/exit foramen stenosis or vascular 'steal'

- Shape and outline of the spinal canal are ideally shown on CT but are also seen simply with MR. It is difficult for MR to distinguish fibrous structures from sclerotic or cortical bone, though it discerns intrathecal contents more readily which is an advantage in identifying intradural tumours. CT is perhaps the preferred choice for investigating canal stenosis.
- Spondylodiscitis (part of SpA), if chronic, may be difficult to discriminate from degenerative disc/vertebral end-plate disease. Fat-suppressed or gadolinium-enhanced sequences may show high signal at the anterior disc vertebral end-plate junctions.

Myelography and CT myelography (using non-ionic contrast)

- Myelographic patterns of abnormality of nerve root entrapment from posterolateral and posterior disc prolapse and spinal stenosis are well-recognized. However, both CT and MR have superceded myelography in most cases.
- Myelography or a combination of CT with radiculopathy is occasionally requested and is useful in patients in whom technical or personal considerations preclude MR examination (about 15% of people).

Screening for infection, malignancy, or metabolic bone disease

- In cases where the history and examination suggest a mechanical condition, but where the clinician wishes to be more confident of excluding an inflammatory condition, an ESR (or plasma viscosity) is suggested.
- A raised ESR would point towards further laboratory investigation.
- An infection screen should include an FBC for anaemia and leucocytosis, CRP, blood and urine cultures. If spinal tuberculosis is suspected a plain CXR should be taken and serial (over 3 days) early morning urine samples taken.
- Urine Bence-Jones proteins and serum immunoglobulin electrophoresis are essential tests in the 'work-up' for myeloma. Serum bone biochemistry and plasma U&E are also important as hypercalcaemia and acute renal impairment have prognostic significance in this condition.
- Serum bone biochemistry may point to an underlying metabolic bone disorder such as Paget's disease or osteomalacia. Bone biochemistry is normal in post-menopausal osteoporosis.
- If osteoporosis is diagnosed a screen for 2° causes should include ESR (and if raised, serum and urinary protein electrophoresis), bone biochemistry, and sex hormones, but also serum 25-hydroxyvitamin D and PTH, TFTs, LFTs, and Cr.

Treatment

- An important therapeutic intervention in the case of acute pain is to take the patient seriously, take a positive view, and in the absence of sinister signs e.g. nerve root pain, urge early mobility.
- Analgesics and antispasmodics can be used in the short term, initially regularly, then as required.
- Physical therapy with graded-activity programmes may be of value, certainly early in disc disease or spondylosis.

- Cord compression 2° to bone collapse from a tumour is an acute emergency and should be discussed immediately with an oncologist or radiotherapist, and a spinal orthopaedic or neurosurgeon.
- Cases with disc prolapse failing to respond to conservative therapy, or cases where there is ongoing or rapidly progressive neurological deficit, should be referred for surgery.
- Available surgical techniques for acute or persistent disc disease include decompression procedures (e.g. nerve root decompression and partial facetectomy), prosthetic intervertebral disc replacement, intradiscal thermocoagulation, and intradiscal steroid injections though evidence for long-term efficacy is lacking for all these procedures.
- Surgery for spinal stenosis is useful for relieving leg neurogenic features but not indicated, even when stenosis proved with MR, if there is no significant leg/sphincter neurocompromise. Surgery is not usually done if the only effect of spinal stenosis is back pain.
- In chronic back pain, aerobic exercises combined with behavioural methods may be more effective than exercise alone and can help reduce 'sickness behaviour'. Methods may also incorporate psychological and social assessment and management.
- The common treatments available for chronic back pain include:
  - analgesics and muscle relaxants
  - antiepileptics/antidepressants for neuropathic pain
  - local anaesthetic/steroid injections
  - acupuncture
  - transcutaneous electrical nerve stimulation (TENS)
  - physiotherapy
  - ergonomic advice
  - multidisciplinary programmes:
    - — counselling
    - — cognitive therapy
    - — education
    - — relaxation
    - — corsets and belts.
- Timely surgery for structural scoliosis (more common in JIA than the general population) can lessen spinal curvature.

Spinal disorders in children and adolescents

Background

- Common conditions in adults such as degenerative back pain and intervertebral disc disease are rare in childhood or adolescence.
- In hospital series upto 85% of referred children have identifiable causes (see Table 2.15) though spinal hypermobility in the context of generalized hypermobility and fibromyalgia has not been adequately addressed.
- Not all presentations are with pain. Some children present with either deformity or neurological symptoms.
- A diagnosis must be firmly established or at least rigorously sought because serious disease can present with few symptoms.

Taking a history

Keep an open mind as to whether a history from the child, parent/s, or 1° care-giver provides the most useful information. There are merits in consulting all of them. The process may be time-consuming.

Table 2.15 Cause of childhood back pain. Experience of an orthopaedic clinic (a review of 233 referrals)

Cause of back pain	Frequency (%)
Non-specific (i.e. no cause found)	32
Scoliosis	21
Spondylolysis/'listhesis (non-trauma)	11
Scheuermann's disease	7
Infection	6
Tumours, e.g. osteoid osteoma	4
Psychogenic	4
Disc prolapse	3
Inflammatory, e.g. spondylarthropathy	3
Trauma (excluding strains)	2
Limb length inequality/biomechanical	2
Renal pain	<1
Rickets	<1
Congenital anomalies	<1

Severity, distribution, and quality of pain

- Pain may be mild even though there is a serious underlying disorder.
- If the pain occurs, or initially occurred, during sport, consider pars interarticularis fractures, spondylolytic spondylolisthesis or Scheuermann's disease (vertebral epiphyseal osteochondritis).
- Persistent pain, unrelieved by rest and disturbing sleep, requires consideration of a bone tumour, bone and/or disc infection, or osteoporotic fracture (steroid-related or juvenile idiopathic osteoporosis (JIO)).
- JIO is rare, occurs between 6 and 13 years of age and is more common in boys. The main differential diagnosis is osteogenesis imperfecta.
- Although uncommon, neurological symptoms such as burning pain, parasthesiae, and weakness in the legs, suggests nerve root irritation.
- Spinal stiffness in a child (typically between 2 and 6 years of age) associated with irritability and a diffusely tender back may be due to infective discitis (though organisms are only found in 50%). In an older child or adolescent (typically 10–15 years of age) and with a less striking history, immobility-related stiffness could represent juvenile enthesitis related arthritis (ERA).

If pain is absent …

Spinal conditions are not always associated with pain. Occasionally a child may present with back deformity or neurological symptoms in the legs alone.

- The history may be non-specific and, for example in a very young child, nothing more than a refusal to walk.
- Scheuermann's disease commonly presents in teenagers with a painless thoracic kyphosis. Pain is more likely to be present if the chondritis is thoracolumbar rather than thoracic. The condition is often asymptomatic.
- Spinal dysraphism (bony abnormality—usually spina bifida, associated with neural anomaly—invariably cord tethering) and spinal cord tumours can often present with neurological leg symptoms/signs alone without back pain. Symptoms may be mild initially.
- Scoliosis is usually pain-free. Pain with scoliosis usually indicates significant underlying pathology. The differential is wide (see Table 2.16).
- The most frequent single cause of a scoliosis in schoolchildren (40%), found from radiographic screening, is pelvic tilt due to leg length inequality.

Table 2.16 Causes of scoliosis in children and adolescents

Structual scolioses (vetebral rotation, vetebral structual change, and loss of normal spinal flexibility)	Idiopathic: infantile (0–3 years); juvenile (3–10 years); adolescent (> 10 years)
	Neuromuscular
	Congenital: failure of vertebral formation, segmentation, or both
	Neurofibromatosis
	Heritable disorders of connective tissue, e.g. osteogenesis imperfecta
	Trauma: fracture; surgical (e.g. post-laminectomy); irradiation
	Spondyloepiphyseal dysplasia
	Metabolic bone disease
	Lumbosacral anomalies (e.g. spondylolytic spondylolisthesis)
	Cervicothoracic anomalies (e.g. cervical fusion (Klippel–Feil))
	Rheumatoid arthritis
	Extraspinal contractures (e.g. post-empyema, post-burns)
Non-structural scolioses (lateral spinal curvature but no vetebral rotation)*	Postural
	Nerve root irritation associated
	Abdominal pain associated (e.g. appendicitis, renal pain)
	Associated with local inflammation
	Spinal infection
	Spinal tumours
	Secondary to leg length discrepancy
	Related to soft-tissue contractures around the hip
	Psychogenic

* It is characteristic of non-structural scolioses that if the underlying cause is successfully dealt with, the scoliosis resolves.

Past developmental, medical, family, and social history

- Ask about milestones in musculoskeletal development. Abnormality or delay might suggest spinal dysraphism or neuromuscular conditions.
- Osteoporosis may be evident from previous fragility fracture— axial or appendicular—or may be intimated from risk factors, e.g. steroid use.
- Previous low back trauma may have been pars interarticularis fractures preceding (the current) vertebral slip or disc prolapse.
- Irradiation (e.g. of previous Wilms' tumour) is a cause of scoliosis.

- Ask about previous TB or immunization against it in patients you think are at risk of TB osteomyelitis.
- Torticollis may be associated with chronic squint, previous trauma (?psychogenic component) and neuroleptic drugs. It can be a sign of an underlying neurological or inflammatory lesion or occurs because of an underlying structural anomaly.
- A history of a heritable disease of connective tissue can often be elicited from the family of a child with structural scoliosis.
- A history of back pain is sometimes elicited from families of children with non-specific back pain. Joint dislocation and multiple soft-tissue musculoskeletal injury (especially overuse) in family members raises the possibility of general hypermobility (either joint hypermobility syndrome or a heritable connective tissue disease, e.g. Marfan syndrome.
- There is often a family history of back pain associated with investigation-negative, non-specific spinal pain (more frequently diagnosed in girls than in boys) that is considered to have a psychogenic component.
- The existence, or child's perception, of social disharmony at home or school is likely to be more important in influencing the impact of back pain rather than a cause of it. Nevertheless in children with non-specific spinal pain or fibromyalgia especially, social conflict resulting in stress and anxiety may be very important in generating symptoms.

Examination

It is best, and certainly ultimately more informative, to undertake the examination only when the child is comfortable with the situation, with their modesty and dignity preserved, and with consent to go ahead after a reassurance that the examination will be stopped if it is painful. With younger children there may be 'an examinable moment', usually after the child has gained confidence in the surroundings and with the situation. Observing the young child whilst playing is a considerate way of starting the examination.

Age-related variations in biomechanical development and gait patterns

- Walking whilst holding a hand or furniture develops by 12 months and normally independent walking by 18 months.
- Until 3 years the stance is broad-based in relation to pelvic width, the knee may not fully extend and the ankle may be plantar flexed at foot-strike.
- Climbing stairs is usually done using alternate feet by age of 3 years.
- Tiptoe walking is not abnormal at first but should disappear by 2 years. If this pattern remains consider spasticity, tethered cord, or muscle weakness.
- Flat feet up to age 5 are normal (a consequence of the distribution of fat and paucity of muscle development). Only investigate if symptomatic.
- Leg alignment often concerns parents. Up until 2 years of age it is normal to have genu varum. From 2–5 years mild genu valgum may occur. Angles of >10° or asymmetry may be associated with underlying disease.
- Regression of motor development is a clue to the presence of disease.

Observation

Observe children unclothed to underwear if possible; initially at play then look from behind. Look for weakness, scoliosis, kyphosis, and swellings.

- The main cause of spinal asymmetry will be scoliosis (see Table 2.16).
- Localized soft tissue swelling may denote soft tissue extension of a spinal tumour though an 'apparent' kyphosis associated with scoliosis is usually a result of spinal rotation.
- In children with neck pain look for a short neck (?Klippel–Fiel) or asymmetric scapulae (Sprengel's deformity: a higher, hypoplastic scapula).
- Adolescent kyphosis may be due to Scheuermann's disease or fractures. Unless there has been steroid use, the former is more likely.
- Note any skin markings such as café-au-lait spots, skin indents (lumbar area) and lumbosacral hair. They may be markers of bony abnormality.
- Note any muscular weakness. With truncal weakness (e.g. DM) the child may have to roll over before getting up from a supine position. Hip girdle weakness may be present in a child unwilling to squat and unable to stand from squatting without exhibiting Gower's sign (unable to stand up from the floor without using hands to push off).

Examine the gait pattern

- Look for asymmetry and a limp.
- Back or leg pain from any cause can give rise to a limp. Also, limp may be the only feature of a serious underlying neurological or bony deformity.
- Asymmetry of shoulder height, transverse posterior skin folds, pelvic tilt, and arm swing may be a clue to spinal pathology.

Spinal examination with the child standing

Examine the whole spine whilst the child is standing. The immature spine is usually far more flexible than an adult's.

- Ask about the presence and site of neck or low back pain during forward flexion, extension, and lateral flexion (and rotation for neck). Experienced examiners should be able to detect significantly limited movements.
- Palpate along the line of (lumbar) spinous processes. An inward step may be caused by spondylolisthesis.
- Palpate any swellings. Lipomata are painless. Soft tissue tumours may be, but are not necessarily, tender and fixed.

Examine the sitting patient

Examine the child who is sitting on the couch, legs hanging over the side.

- This is the best way to elicit pain from posterior vertebral structure pathology in thoracic or lumbar segments (e.g. pars osteoid osteoma, pars fracture). Combine extension and rotation movements. Ask if the pain is worse on one side than the other.

Examine the supine patient

Examine the child or adolescent when supine. Look for leg length discrepancy, lower leg asymmetry, and do a neurological examination.

- Measure and determine actual or apparent leg length discrepancy. True leg length discrepancy is a cause of non-structural scoliosis. Apparent leg length discrepancy/pelvic tilts can occur to compensate for scoliosis caused by spinal lesions.
- Different foot or leg sizes/appearances are a non-specific sign of spinal dysraphism.
- Hip and sacroiliac examination should be done routinely in children with low back pain. Tests for dural irritation and neurological examination are essential (see section on Low back pain and disorders in adults, pp.74–87).
- Though limb pain, weakness and other neurological symptoms occur, the majority of children with intradural tumours have none of these features. A normal examination does not rule out serious pathology.

Examine the prone patient

- Palpate over the spinous processes, interspinous spaces, paracentrally between spinous processes (over facet joints) and in the sacroiliac area.
- Diffuse tenderness may only be a reflection of muscle spasm and its extensive mechanical effect. Where there are isolated areas of tenderness feel for skin warmth, as this may be a site of infection.

Investigations

Radiographs

- Radiographs have a characteristic appearance in certain cases of bone tumour but may also, in some cases, be normal (see Table 2.17).
- A normal bone scan rules out most serious pathology.
- A widened interpedicular distance on an AP film is a sign of meningomyelocele or spinal dysraphism, also of an intraspinal mass.
- Posterior vertebral scalloping on a lateral radiograph is most obviously seen in lumbar or cervical spines, most prominent in association with lesions occurring in childhood and most commonly due to spinal tumours, neurofibromatosis, osteogenesis imperfecta, Ehlers–Danlos, and Marfan syndrome.
- Spondylolysis/pars fractures may be visible on lateral X-rays but are best characterized by oblique films. Associated internal disc derangement or radiculopathy is best characterized using MR.
- Appearances of Scheuermann's disease (multiple irregular vertebral endplates, with anterior ring epiphyseal fragmentation and vertebral wedging) are an occasional incidental X-ray finding.
- Radiographs of the neck may show a degree of cervical fusion (Klippel–Feil). Suspect hypermobility in non-affected segments and investigate C1/C2 with MR if there are high cervical pain or myelopathic symptoms.

Table 2.17 Radiographic features of spinal tumours in children (see also Table 20.7)

Tumour type	Notable clinical features and radiological appearances
Osteochondroma	Has the appearance of an exostosis
Osteoid osteoma	Radiographs often normal. Bone scintigraphy will localize lesion and CT sharply define it
Osteoblastoma	Lytic with central ossification on radiograph. Can metastasize
Aneurysmal bone cyst	Lucent lesion with central trabeculae on radiographs. MR important to document soft-tissue expansion
Langerhan's cell histiocytosis (eosinophilic granuloma)	Either solitary, polyostotic, or associated with systemic illness. Lytic lesion can cause solitary vertebral collapse, even collapse of adjacent bones. Used to be called histiocytosis X
Myeloma	Rare in children. Lytic lesions on radiographs. Distribution of lesions can be shown with bone scintigraphy but use as adjunct to radiographs
Ewing's sarcoma	Age 5–20 usually. 'Moth-eaten' destruction of bone on radiograph
Lymphoma	Sclerotic ('ivory') vertebra on film
Osteosarcoma	Mixed lytic/sclerotic appearance on radiographs
Metastases	Most likely are from leukaemia or neuroblastoma
Intra- and extramedullary tumours	Delay in diagnosis common. Up to 50% have abnormal films: widened spinal canal, pedicle erosions, scalloping of vertebral bodies. MR usually characterizes the lesion

- Bone scintigraphy is sensitive to detect spinal bony abnormality and a –ve test rules out most subtle lesions e.g. osteoid osteomas.
- Consider SIJ radiographs and MR in patients with prominent immobility-related low back pain and stiffness (commonly due spondylarthropathy-related conditions).

Investigating scoliosis

- The cause of painful scoliosis must be determined. Consider MR or CT of any localized area of pain. Idiopathic scoliosis is asymptomatic and is a diagnosis of exclusion.
- Mild idiopathic scoliosis (5–10°) can be determined on a posteroanterior thoracolumbar radiograph and is relatively common in the school population (7%). A scoliosis of > 20° occurs in 1 in 500 people and is three to four times more common in girls than boys.
- In 10–20% of those with a trunk inclination of > 5° , the scoliosis progresses at least a further 5° . Most have a non-progressive scoliosis.

Laboratory investigations

Laboratory investigations should be sought if infection, inflammation or malignancy is considered (see section on low back pain and disorders in adults).

Pelvic, groin, and thigh pain

Anatomy

Anatomy of the pelvis and hip region

- The bony pelvis consists of two inominate bones (ilium above the acetabulum and ischium below it) that articulate with each other at the anterior symphysis pubis and posteriorly with the sacrum at the SIJs.
- SIJs are initially synovial but become fibrous with age. A few degrees of rotation can be demonstrated in children and young adults.
- Strong ligaments stabilize the posterior pelvis through sacroinominate, lumbo(L5)–sacral, and lumbo(L5)–iliac attachments.
- The symphysis pubis is a cartilagenous joint and normally does not move.
- When standing, weight is transferred through the head of the femur that is stablized in the acetabulum and its surrounding fibrous labrum by strong pericapsular ligaments.
- The ligamentum teres crosses the hip joint and carries blood vessels to the head of the femur in children and young adults. In old age, blood supply is largely via vessels that enter the femoral neck.
- Bursae are associated with gluteus maximus at its insertion: one behind, and separating it from, the greater trochanter; the other in front of the bone separating gluteus maximus from part of the origin of vastus lateralis.
- The ischial bursa separates gluteus maximus from the ischial tuberosity and can become inflamed from frictional injury.

Anatomy of pelvic musculature

- Three groups of muscles move the hip joint: gluteals, flexor muscles, and the adductor group.
- The major gluteal group muscles are:
  - gluteus maximus (L5, S1/2): arises mainly from ilium and sacrum, swathes down posteriolaterally and inserts into the posterior femur (20% of it) but mainly into the lateral tensor fasciae latae. It extends and externally rotates the hip (hamstrings also extend the hip).
  - gluteus medius (L4/5, S1): lies deeper and more lateral. It inserts into the lateral greater trochanter and abducts and internally rotates the hip.
  - piriformis, obdurator internus, and quadratus femoris arise deep in the pelvis and insert into the posterior greater trochanter. All externally rotate the hip.
- The major hip flexor, psoas major (L2/3), is a massive muscle that arises from the lateral part of the vertebrae and intervertebral discs (T12–L5) and lateral processes of the lumbar vertebrae. It runs anteriorly over the iliac rim, across the pelvis, under the inguinal ligament, and inserts into the lesser trochanter. Iliacus (L2–L4) arises from the 'inside' of the iliac blade, passes under the inguinal ligament medially to the lesser trochanter. Both flex but psoas also internally rotates the hip.

- Psoas is enveloped in a fascial sheath. Retroperitoneal or spinal infection which tracks along soft tissue planes sometimes involves the psoas sheath and can cause inflammation in the psoas bursa, which separates the muscle from the hip joint which it overlies.
- All adductor muscles arise from the pubis or ischiopubic rami. Adductor longus and gracilis are the most superficial, arise most medially—from the pubis—and insert into the femoral shaft and pes anserinus ('goose's foot') below the knee, respectively. Adductor magnus (L4/5) is the largest of the deeper adductors and inserts into the length of the medial femoral shaft.
- Adductors stabilize movement about the hip towards the end of the stance phase of the gait. Body weight is transferred onto one leg during this action, thus adductors need to be strong, especially for running.

Functional anatomy of the hip

- With a flexed knee the limit of hip flexion is about 135°.
- Hip extension (at 30°), and internal (at 30–35°) and external (at 45–55°) rotation is limited by strong, pericapsular ligaments.
- Abduction is limited to 45–50° by contact between the greater trochanter and acetabular labrum rim and adduction to 20–30° (leg swung across other) with a fixed pelvis. These are adult ranges.
- Greater femoral neck anteversion (angulation of neck compared to a line drawn through the femoral condyles in the coronal plane) allows greater internal rotation of the hip (and reduced external rotation). Tibial torsion can compensate but often this and hip anteversion results in a toe-in gait. Femoral neck retroversion (if the angle is posterior to the femoral intercondylar plane) allows greater external rotation of the hip, usually resulting in a toe-out gait (see Fig. 2.21).
- Normally infants have more anteversion than older children or adults (30–40° at age 2 compared with 8–15° at age > 18).

Neuroanatomy

- The femoral nerve is formed from L2–L4 nerve roots and supplies mainly muscles of the quadriceps group and some deeper hip adductors.
- With contributions from L4–S3 roots, nerves from the plexus converge at the inferior border of the piriformis to form the sciatic nerve. This is at a foramen formed by the ilium (above and lateral), sacrum (medial), sacrospinous ligament (below), and sacrotuberous ligament (posteromedial).
- In about 10% of people the sciatic nerve divides before exiting the pelvis. In some a branch exits above the piriformis muscle. Nerve entrapment and trauma from intramuscular injections at this site is recognized (Piriformis syndrome).

Taking a history

Age

Age is a risk factor for some conditions:

- Congenital hip dislocation is common (prevalence 1:500) and more so in girls vs. boys (8:1). It should be considered in toddlers if there is delay in motor milestones or pain on 'weight-bearing'.
- The commonest cause of hip pain in children aged 2–12 years is transient synovitis (unilateral, self-limiting). The differential diagnosis includes Legg–Calvé–Perthes' disease (osteonecosis of femoral head) and Lyme or post-streptococcal arthritis.
- Legg–Calvé–Perthes' disease (age 3–12 years) is four to five times more common in boys and bilateral in 10–20% of cases.
- Slipped capital epiphysis is rare in children aged <8 and > 16 years. It is associated with obesity and endocrine disorders (4% are hypothyroid).
- Unless there has been previous hip disease (e.g. osteonecrosis, synovitis), trauma, or a long-standing biomechanical abnormality
- (e.g. epiphyseal dysplasia, heritable disease of connective tissue), hip osteoarthritis (OA) is uncommon in adults <55.
- Paget's disease of bone is rare in adults <50.

Distribution and type of bone and soft tissue pain

- All mechanical lesions of the lumbar spine can result in referred pain around the pelvis/thighs. It is often bilateral, localizes poorly, and is aching in nature.
- Lateral pelvic pain is often referred from the lumbosacral spine. If pain localizes well (i.e. patient points) to the greater trochanter, it may be due to trochanteric bursitis, enthesitis, or meralgia parasthetica (see Table 2.18).
- Hip joint pain is felt in the groin, though it can be located deep in the buttock when ischial bursitis and sacroiliac pain should also be considered. It may be referred distally to the anteromedial thigh and knee.
- Groin pain on weight-bearing suggests hip pathology such as synovitis; osteonecrosis or OA but is not specific. Tendonitis of adductor longus, osteitis pubis, a femoral neck stress fracture (4% of all stress fractures), osteoid osteoma, or psoas bursitis can give similar symptoms.
- Bone pathology typically gives unremitting pain. Sleep is often disturbed.
- Pain from deep musculoskeletal pelvic structures is typically poorly localized though can be extremely severe. If the pain appears to be 'catastrophic' consider pelvic bone disease (tumours, infection, Paget's disease, osteomalacia, osteoporotic fracture), or an unstable pelvis (chronic osteitis pubis with diastasis/laxity of the symphysis pubis and SIJs).
- Enthesitis and osteitis pubis associated with spondylarthropathy (SpA) are probably under-recognized.

Table 2.18 Patterns of pain around the proximal leg and their major causes

Pattern of pain	Causes
Pain in buttock and posterior thighs	Referred pain from: lumbar spine e.g. facet, OA, spondylolisthesis; SIJ inflammation; lower lumbar nerve root irritation; sciatic nerve entrapment (piriformis syndrome)
	Localized pain: ischial bursitis/enthesitis or fracture; coccidynia
	Diffuse muscular pain/stiffness: myositis or PMR
	Paget's or other bone lesion of sacrum
Lateral pelvic pain	Referred from lumbosacral spine
	Trochanteric bursitis/enthesitis
	Gluteus medius tear
	Lateral hip joint pain, e.g. osteophyte
Groin pain	Hip disease, e.g. OA, osteonecrosis, synovitis
	Psoas bursitis
	Adductor tendonitis, osteitis pubis
	Pelvic enthesitis
	Paget's disease (pelvis or femur)
	Femoral neck or pubic ramus fracture
	Hernia
Anterior or medial pain	Referred from: lumbar spine, e.g. facet OA, thigh spondylolisthesis; upper lumbar nerve root; hip joint, femoral neck, psoas bursa
	Myositis, PMR, diabetic amyotrophy
	Meralgia parasthetica (anterolateral)
	Adductor tendonitis, osteitis pubis
	Ischaemia (claudication)
	Lymph nodes

- Aching in the back of the legs after standing is typical of, but not specific for, spondylolisthesis.
- Sacroiliac pain and stiffness radiates to the buttocks and posterior thighs.

Pain in a muscular distribution

- Diffuse pain in the buttocks and thighs occurs in polymyalgia rheumatica (PMR). It is often sudden or subacute in onset, associated with stiffness, and may give similar symptoms to those caused by sacroiliitis but invariably occurs for the first time in a much older age group.
- Pain from autoimmune myositis is unlikely to be confined to pelvic musculature or be unilateral, but should be considered where acute or subacute onset diffuse pelvic girdle/thigh pain accompanies weakness.

Quality and distribution of nerve pain

- Nerve root pain is often clearly defined and sharp. It may be burning in quality and is often accompanied by numbness or parasthesiae. L5 or S1 lesions generally cause pain below the knee though can cause posterior thigh pain. L1–L3 root lesions can cause pain in the anteromedial thigh.
- Pain with parasthesiae on the anterolateral part of the thigh may be due to entrapment of the lateral cutaneous nerve of the thigh under the lateral part of the inguinal ligament (meralgia paraesthetica). Symptoms may be referred to this area with L2 or L3 nerve root lesions as these roots are from where the nerve originates (see Fig. 2.11).
- Diabetics with uncontrolled hyperglycaemia are at risk of amyotrophy. Acute unilateral or bilateral thigh pain with muscle wasting occurs. It should not be misdiagnosed as PMR, in which weakness/wasting does not occur, or autoimmune myositis.
- Soccer players are at risk of adductor tendonitis (often an adductor apophysitis) and osteitis pubis owing to substantial mechanical forces placed on pelvic structures during running and kicking.
- Though hip fractures usually present obviously and acutely, be aware that they can present subacutely with patients still able to walk (particularly stress fractures and in the elderly).

Previous trauma, low back, and musculoskeletal problems

- Previous trauma/disease causing permanent deformity of any lumbosacral or hip joint structure can be considered a risk for further trouble (see Table 2.19).
- Multiparity is a risk for osteitis pubis, sacroiliac, and pelvic pain.
- Trochanteric bursitis may coexist with referred back pain.
- Tears of the gluteus medius can occur at its greater trochanter insertion and give similar symptoms to those caused by bursitis.
- Historically, tailors were at risk of ischial bursitis because of sitting on the floor continually crossing and uncrossing their legs, which causes friction irritation of soft tissues overlying the ischial tuberosity.

Examination

The reader is referred to the sequence of examination for the low back including sacroiliac and lower limb neurological examination (see pp. 80–83). Always consider lower spinal, muscle, or neurological pathology when assessing weakness and pain around the pelvis.

Observation and palpation

For observation and palpation the patient should be supine on a couch:

- Look for leg length discrepancy (hip disease, scoliosis) and a leg resting in external rotation (hip fracture).
- Psoriasis over the knees might be associated with sacroiliitis.

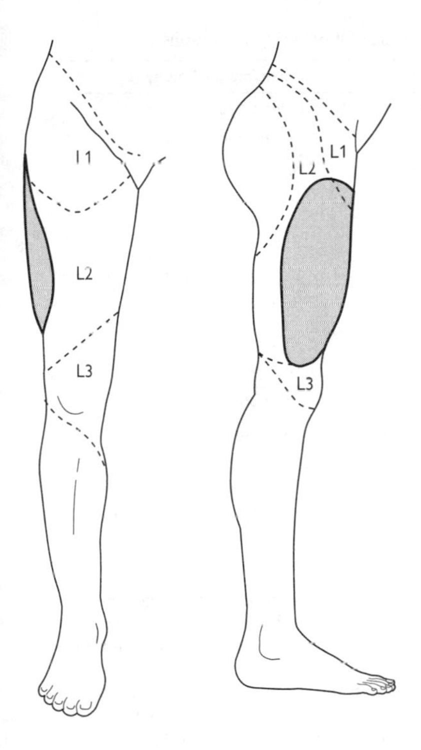

Fig. 2.11 The approximate areas within which sensory changes may be found in lesions of the lateral cutaneous nerve of the thigh (hatched area) and high lumbar radiculopathy (broken line). Shaded area-sensory symptoms distribution from Meralgia Parasthetica.

Table 2.19 Risk factors for painful pelvic or hip lesions

Risk factor	Pelvic/hip pathology
Mechanical abnormality of the low back	Referred pain
	Trochanteric bursitis
Mechanical abnormality of the hip (e.g. Perthes', slipped epiphysis, epiphyseal dysplasia, Paget's)	Hip OA
Corticosteroid use	Osteoporotic fracture
	Osteonecrosis of the femoral head
Autoimmune rheumatic disease (e.g.RA, JIA, AS)	Synovitis hip
	Secondary OA of the hip
	Pyogenic arthritis of the hip
	Osteoporotic fracture
Maternal history of hip fracture; low body mass index; low bone mass; falls	Osteoporotic hip fracture
Multiple pregnancies	Osteitis pubis (± pelvic instability)
Soccer players	Adductor tendonitis/apophysitis
	Osteitis pubis

- Swelling in the groin may be a hernia (?reducible or cough impulse), lipomata (soft/non-tender/diffuse), a saphenous varix, or lymphadenopathy (hard/rubbery and invariably mobile). A hip joint effusion cannot be felt.
- Tenderness over the hip joint in the groin is not specific for joint pathology (the joint is deep, muscles and psoas bursa overlie it).
- If the groin is very tender with slight touch, consider hip fracture or infection. Hyperpathia (and allodynia) is consistent with algodystrophy.
- Numbness over the anterolateral thigh suggests meralgia paraesthetica (see Fig. 2.11).
- The adductor longus tendon can be palpated at its insertion at the pubic tubercle and distally along the upper medial thigh. The pubic tubercle is found by palpating slowly and lightly downwards from umbilicus over the bladder until bone is reached.
- Pain from osteitis pubis or adductor apophysitis is often ↑ with abdominal rectus contraction (ask the patient to slowly lift their head and shoulders off the couch keeping your finger on the pubic tubercle).

Hip examination

The patient is supine. Tests generally help to discriminate intra-from extra-articular disease but not causes of intra-articular disease:

- Measure and determine actual or apparent leg length discrepancy: measure from the anterior superior iliac spine to the medial tibial malleolus then, by flexing hips and knees, the site of shortening should become apparent.

- A fixed loss of extension is a sign of intra-articular hip disease. The patient flexes the hip and knee on one side until normal lumbar lordosis flattens out (confirmed by feeling pressure on your hand placed under their lumbar spine during the manoeuvre). If the other hip flexes simultaneously, it suggests hip extension loss on that side (Thomas' test).
- Using the patella or tibial tubercle as pointers, test the rotational hip range in extension by rotating the straightened legs holding the heels.
- Rotational movements are also tested by lifting the leg, flexed 90° at the knee, and swinging the foot out (internal rotation) or in (external rotation). Hip flexion can be tested in this position too. Patients without intra-articular pathology should have a pain-free range of movement.
- Rotational ranges in hip flexion and extension may differ between left and right in an individual. Also, variations in femoral neck anteversion contribute to variations in rotation range.
- To test hip abduction/adduction, fix the pelvis to avoid pelvic tilt by placing one hand firmly over the iliac crest. Occasionally, pain at the end of abduction or internal rotation occurs with a bony block (solid 'end-feel'). In an older patient this might suggest impingement of a marginal joint osteophyte.
- Barlow's manoeuvre checks for congenital dislocation of the hips in babies. Flex and adduct the hips exerting an axial force into the posterior 'acetabulum' to demonstrate posterior dislocation.
- Greater retroversion (allowing excessive hip external rotation) usually occurs in cases of slipped femoral epiphysis. External rotation is accentuated when the hip is flexed. The slip (usually inferoposterior) is thought to occur in association with a period of rapid growth.

Muscle activation tests

Specific muscle activation against resistance can be used to elicit pain, but results need to be interpreted cautiously in the context of known hip disease:

- Hip adduction against resistance (sliding their leg inwards towards the other against your hand) reproducing pain is a sensitive test for adductor longus tendonitis but may be positive in osteitis pubis, hip joint lesions, and other soft tissue lesions in the adductor muscles.
- Test psoas by resisted hip flexion in slight internal rotation. Psoas bursitis or infection tracking along the psoas sheath is likely to give intense pain with minimal resistance.
- Hip abduction (sliding the leg outwards against your hand) may be particularly painful in cases of gluteus medius tears but also in trochanteric bursitis or intra-articular pathology.

Palpate posterolateral structures

Ask the patient to lie on their side and palpate the posterolateral structures (see Fig. 2.12):

- Tenderness over the greater trochanter is usually well-localized although it may be anterior or posterolateral to the trochanter and refers a small way down the leg.

- The ischial tuberosity and its overlying bursa lie at the apex of the buttock.
- The soft tissues overlying the point where the sciatic nerve exits the pelvis is found midway between the ischial spine and the greater trochanter. There may be tenderness as a result of soft tissue lesions or trauma causing sciatic nerve entrapment (painful foot drop—piriformis syndrome).
- A tender coccyx (coccidynia) can be palpated in this position. It can also be palpated and the sacrococcygeal joint moved from a bidigital examination, though this requires the index finger to be placed inside the rectum, the thumb outside, the two digits then holding the joint.

Investigations

Radiographs

An AP radiograph of the pelvis is a good initial screening test in patients with pelvic, hip, or thigh pain. AP and lateral lumbar spine films may be warranted.

- The pelvis is a common site of involvement in myeloma, metastatic malignancy, and Paget's disease of bone.
- Established, but often not early, sacroiliitis can be ruled out. The main differential diagnoses of the causes of sacroiliitis are: AS, psoriatic or reactive arthritis, enteric arthropathy including Whipple's disease, brucellosis and other infections, hyperparathyroidism and osteitis condensans ilii (sclerosis of the SIJ on the lower iliac side).
- Widening of the symphysis in children may be a sign of congenital disorders of development (e.g. epispadias, achondrogenesis, chondrodysplasias, hypophosphatasia), trauma and hyperparathyroidism.
- Widening of the symphysis pubis, osteitis pubis (bone resorption and sclerosis) and osteitis condensans ilii are signs associated with chronic pelvic pain in multiparous women.
- General osteopenia may be reported and is a risk factor for general low bone mass measured by densitometry; however, it is not a sensitive or specific indicator of osteoporosis (e.g. may be osteomalacia or rickets).
- Regional osteoporosis confined to the femur is non-specific but may reflect hip synovitis, infection, or transient osteoporosis of the hip (rare).
- Early synovitis and infection may be demonstrated through subtle radiological signs such as joint space widening and change in soft tissue fat planes.
- A 'frogs' legs' (lateral) view of the hip shows the anterior and posterior femoral head more clearly than an AP view (useful in early osteonecrosis/Perthes', slipped epiphysis).

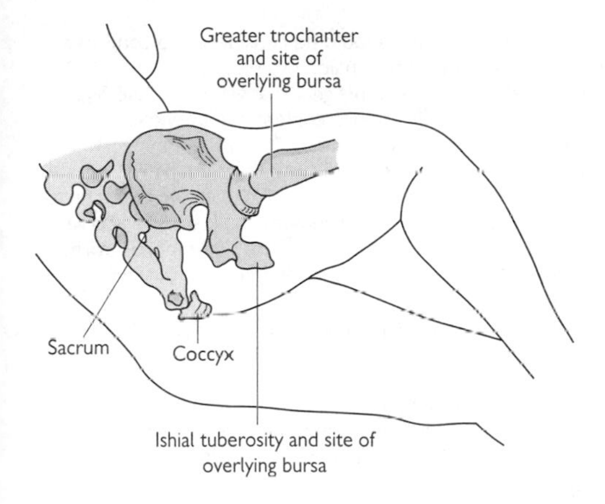

Fig. 2.12 Bony anatomy of the posterior hip and pelvis, showing the position in which lesions around the greater trochanter and ischial bursa can be palpated

- The acetabulae are best visualized on 45° oblique views (acetebular fractures can be missed on a conventional AP view).
- 'Stork' views of the symphysis pubis (standing on one leg) are useful for confirming diastasis of the joint.

Diagnostic ultrasound

- US is a sensitive and simple way of confirming a hip joint effusion. Fluid can be aspirated for culture relatively easily and an assessment of the extent of synovial thickening can be made.
- Tendon damage in the groin area should be identifiable with US alone (guided steroid injection can then be done if necessary) but MR may be needed either to characterize pathology further or rule out joint pathology.

Bone scintigraphy

Bone scintigraphy is a useful screening test though is often nonspecific:

- Characteristic, though non-specific, patterns of bone scan abnormality are recognized in the hip/pelvic area. The following conditions can be recognized: sacroiliitis, bone malignancy, myeloma, Paget's disease, hip fracture, femoral head osteonecrosis, osteoid osteoma, OA and synovitis of the hip, osteitis pubis/adductor apophysitis (requires special seated 'ring' view), and bursitis/enthesitis at the greater trochanter.
- Bone scintigraphy is a useful investigation in children and adolescents as a screening investigation if radiology is normal and symptoms remain.

CT and MR

- CT/MR of the high lumbar region should be considered to confirm a nerve root lesion causing groin/thigh pain.
- Specific patterns of X-ray attenuation/signal change around the SIJs occur in sacroiliitis with CT/MR, though current and previous inflammation cannot easily be distinguished.
- A suspicion of bony malignancy from radiographs of the pelvis requires further characterization. CT is the technique of choice for characterizing bone lesions around the hip such as femoral neck stress fracture, osteoid osteoma, or other bone tumours. CT may give more information about the lesion (and is valuable in 'guided biopsy') but MR is useful in checking for pelvic visceral lesions.
- MR is the technique of choice if hip infection or osteonecrosis is suspected. In adults, patterns of signal change have been correlated with prognosis.
- During a single examination the pattern of hip synovitis (vascularity and thickness), cartilage loss, and subchondral bone erosion can be documented. This is particularly useful in children with JIA.

Laboratory investigations

- ESR and CRP may be normal in inflammatory SIJ, lumbar vertebral disc, and pelvic enthesis disorders.
- PMR is invariably associated with an acute phase response.
- Myeloma is unlikely if the ESR is normal.
- A high ALP is typically associated with an acute phase response, although association with pelvic pain in the elderly might suggest Paget's disease.
- ANA and RF are unlikely to help diagnostically.
- Major metabolic bone disease such as osteomalacia and hyperparathyroidism is usually excluded by a normal serum calcium and phosphate.

Treatment

Treatment of spinal and neuropathic pain is covered in the section on Low back pain and disorders in adults (pp.74–87).

- Simple and NSAID analgesia may be required for a number of the conditions described above, particularly OA, hip synovitis, and tendon inflammation.
- Physiotherapy and rehabilitation play a vital and early part in management, maintaining mobility, preventing tissue contracture, and restrengthening/stabilizing the lower back, pelvis, and hip.
- Either physiotherapists or podiatrists may help in accurately evaluating back and lower limb biomechanics. Asymmetry and muscular imbalance may be modifiable relatively simply with foot orthotics, for example.
- Steroid injections may be important in the following conditions:
  - meralgia parasthetica
  - osteitis pubis
  - trochanteric bursitis/enthesitis
  - ischial bursitis/enthesitis
  - adductor tendonitis
  - coccydinia

- hip synovitis (under imaging guidance)
- sacroiliitis—in intractable pain and under X-ray or US guidance.
- Injection techniques are covered at the end of this chapter, p.148.

Surgery

- When the hip has been damaged by an inflammatory arthritis or OA the principal surgical intervention is joint replacement. Osteotomy has been mainly superceded by more reliable replacement.
- Surgical synovectomy of the hip is a difficult procedure and opening the hip carries a risk of avascular necrosis. This procedure is very rarely done.
- Excision arthroplasty is only really necessary where infection or poor bone stock make reconstruction unwise. Power is often greatly reduced and even the previously fit young patient will often require two sticks as walking aids.
- In children in particular, it is important to assess spinal and knee disease, especially contractures, before embarking on hip surgery as the 1° cause for flexion deformities or hip damage may be at these levels.

Knee pain

Anatomy of the knee

- The knee extends, flexes and also rotates.
- The main extensor quadriceps consists of four muscle segments—rectus femoris, vastus lateralis, medialis, and intermedius—which converge to form a tendon containing the patella which then inserts into the tibia. Rectus femoris arises from the pelvis and vastus muscles from the upper femur.
- The hamstring muscles (biceps femoris, semitendinosus, semimembranosus) all arise from the ischial tuberosity and flex the knee. Biceps femoris inserts around the fibular head. The other two muscles insert into the tibia on the medial side and can externally rotate the femur.
- In the knee the femoral condyles articulate within semicircular fibrocartilage menisci on the tibial condyles (see Fig 2.13). Only the peripheral 10–30% of the menisci is vascular and innervated and can potentially repair.
- As the knee approaches full extension the femur internally rotates on the tibia (biceps femoris action) tightening each pair of ligaments relative to each other (see Fig. 2.13). This configuration confers maximum stability.
- As flexion is initiated a small amount of femoral external rotation on the tibia occurs. This 'unlocking' is done by popliteus—a muscle which arises from the posterior surface of the tibia below. It passes up obliquely across the back of the knee and inserts, via a cord-like tendon, into the lateral femoral condyle. The tendon partly lies within the knee joint capsule.
- Grooves on the femoral condyle articular surfaces allow tight congruity with the anterior horns of the menisci when the knee is extended. If full extension—and this optimal articulation configuration—is lost then articular cartilage degeneration invariably follows (important in inflammatory arthritis).
- The cruciate ligaments are the principal joint stabilizers. The anterior cruciate attaches above to the inside of the lateral femoral condyle and below to the tibia in front of the tibial spines though a slip attaches to the anterior horn of the lateral meniscus. Its main role is to control and contain the amount of knee rotation when the joint is flexed.
- The posterior cruciate attaches above to the inside of the medial femoral condyle. Below it attaches in a (posterior) groove between tibial condyles. Its main role is to stabilize the joint by preventing forward displacement of the femur relative to the tibia when the knee is flexed.
- The cruciates are extra-articular and are covered by a layer of vascular synovium. Bleeding usually accompanies disruption.
- The tibial or medial collateral ligament (MCL) has superficial and deep layers (see Fig. 2.14). It stabilizes the knee against valgus stresses mostly during flexion. The superficial MCL overlies, and moves relative to, the deep part and is separated from it by a bursa. The lower part of the superficial MCL is covered by the long adductors, gracilis,

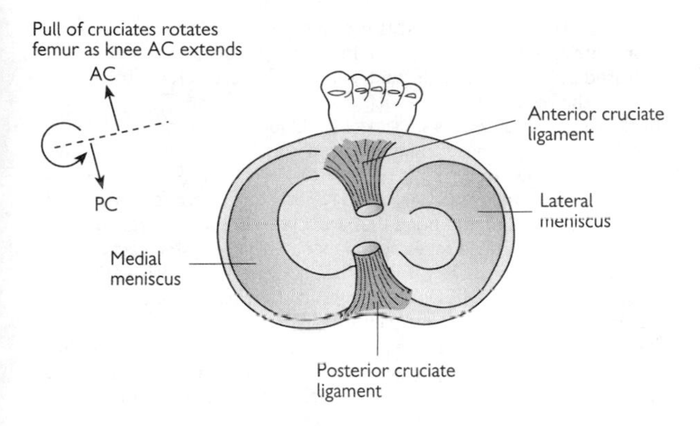

Fig. 2.13 Axial section of the right knee joint (looking down on the tibial plateau, where the foot is fixed on the floor). The femoral condyles articulate within the menisci. As the knee extends the cruciate ligaments tighten and pull the femoral condyles acting to internally rotate the femur through the last few degrees of extension. The knee therefore 'locks' and is stable when the leg is straight

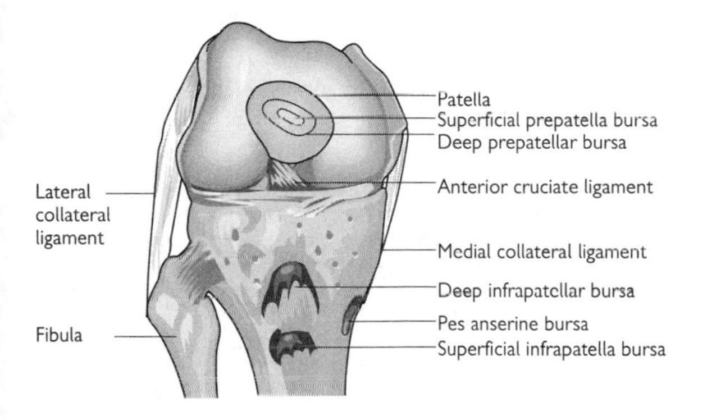

Fig. 2.14 Anterior knee structures

semitendinosus, and sartorius, as they merge (as the pes anserinus) before inserting into the tibia. The MCL and pes anserinus are separated by the anserine bursa. Deeper MCL fibres attach to, and stabilize, the medial meniscus.

- The fibular or lateral collateral ligament (LCL) joins the lateral femoral condyle to the fibular head and is separated from it by a bursa. It stabilizes the knee on its lateral side. It has no meniscal attachment. A small bursa separates it from the overlapping tendon insertion of biceps femoris.
- The patella is a sesamoid bone that articulates in the femoral condylar groove and makes quadriceps action more efficient. Patella articular facet configuration can vary, though not convincingly consistently with any specific condition; however, congenital bi/tripartite patellae are associated with anterior knee pain.
- The strongest force on the patella is from vastus lateralis (see Fig. 2.15). Mechanical factors which increase the ratio of lateral to medial forces during patella tracking such as a wide pelvis, a more lateral origin of vastus lateralis, femoral neck anteversion, external tibial torsion and a weak vastus medialis are risk factors for patella maltracking and anterior knee pain.
- There are bursae (see Fig. 2.14) between the quadriceps tendon and the femur (suprapatellar), the patellar tendon and tibial tubercle (deep infrapatellar), and overlying the patella (prepatellar) and patellar tendon insertion (superficial infrapatellar). The suprapatellar bursa communicates with the knee joint and large joint effusions invariably fill it.
- Posteriorly, bursae separate each of the heads of gastrocnemius (which arise from femoral condyles) from the joint capsule. The bursae communicate with the knee joint and can fill from joint effusions.

Taking a history

Ask about the site of pain

Try to establish whether pain is from articular, soft tissue, or anterior knee structures. Is it referred pain?

- Bursa, tendon, and most ligament lesions cause well-localized pain.
- Localized tibiofemoral joint line pain suggests meniscal pathology.
- Localized medial knee pain has a number of possible causes: MCL tear or chronic inflammation (calcification of MCL origin termed the Pellegrini–Stieda phenomenon), medial meniscus tear, meniscal cyst, anserine tendonitis, bursitis, or enthesitis (?semimembranosus insertion).
- Enthesitis of structures at their insertion to the patella margins can result in considerable pain.
- Overuse in runners and cyclists can cause localized inflammation and pain of the iliotibial band (ITB) or its underlying bursa over the lateral femoral condyle (as the band moves across the bone as the knee flexes).
- Anterior pain in children, adolescents, and young adults invariably suggests an underlying mechanical abnormality. In older adults the commonest cause is patellofemoral OA (see Table 2.20).
- Anterior knee pain may be referred from the hip or L3 nerve root. Hip pain is an aching pain, root pain is sharp often with parasthesiae.

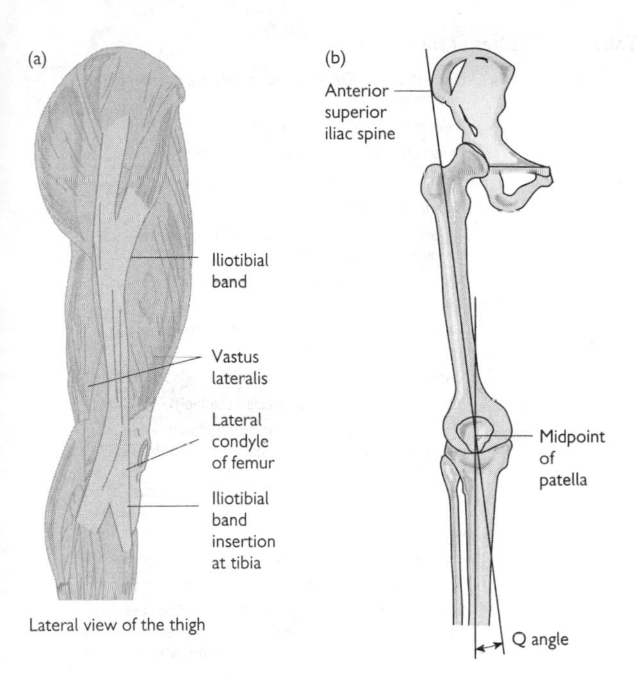

Fig. 2.15 (a) The iliotibial band. (b) The patella Q angle (normal values—men 10°, women 15°)

- Posterior knee pain associated with 'a lump' is often due to synovitis in the posterior knee compartment with popliteal cyst formation (Baker's cyst).

Ask about injury

Knee injuries are common, the most significant is anterior cruciate injury. Ask about injury and whether the knee feels unstable or 'gives way'.

- Anterior cruciate injuries are invariably associated with a haemarthrosis, thus a painful effusion will have occurred immediately. Meniscus tears can cause immediate pain but synovitis and swelling are delayed for about 6 h.
- Patients may volunteer that the knee 'keeps going out'. This feeling may be the pivot shift phenomenon caused by reduced anterior cruciate stability against a valgus stress as the knee is flexing.
- Anterior cruciate and MCL injuries often coexist (they are attached). Ask about medial knee pain originally and subsequently.

Table 2.20 Causes of anterior knee pain

Commonly in adults	Patellofemoral OA (look for mechanical factors and generalized OA)
	Referred hip pain, e.g. hip OA
	Referred pain from L3 nerve root irritation
Specific to children and adolescents	Referred pain from the hip, e.g. slipped femoral epiphysis
	Bi-/tripartite patella
	Synovial plicae (synovial shelf clicking over femoral condyle on knee flexion)
	Recurrent patellar dislocation (tissue laxity, patella alta, trauma)
	Osteochondritis at patellar lower pole—overuse injury in jumping sports*
	Osteochondritis of tibial tubercle (Osgood–Schlatter's)
	Non-specific ('chondromalacia patellae')
Causes at any age	Mechanical factors (?patellar maltracking): wide pelvis, femoral anteversion, external tibial torsion; specific strengthening of lateral structures, e.g.iliotibial band syndrome; weakness or injury of vastus medialis or medial knee structures; tissue laxity, e.g. benign joint hypermobility syndrome
	Osteochondritis dissecans of patella (average age 18)
	Enthesitis at patellar margins (may be part of SpA)
	Bursitis (prepatellar, superficial/deep infrapatellar): gout (very rare in children unless inherited metabolic deficiency); autoimmune rheumatic disease; infection
	Tear/cyst of anterior meniscal horn
	Patellar fracture
	Fat pad syndrome (recurrent retropatella tendon pain with swelling)

*Sinding–Larsen–Johansson disease.

Ask about knee locking

Knee locking is a mechanical effect of disruption of normal articulation by 'loose bodies'.

- Suspect meniscus damage in the middle aged or if the patient plays a lot of sport. A meniscus tear is the commonest cause of the knee locking.
- In adolescents, locking may be due to a tear in a discoid meniscus (>98% lateral). The morphologically abnormal discs are prone to degeneration.
- Chondral fragments (from osteochondritis dissecans lesions) can cause locking; the condition is commonest in the 5–20 year age group (boys > girls).
- Synovial chondromatosis is a rare cause.
- Some patients with anterior knee pain describe the knee locking or giving way. This is due to reflex quadriceps inhibition rather than true instability.

Ask about the initial onset of pain

- Acute pain is usual with injuries of cruciates and vertical meniscal tears.
- Acute onset pain without trauma (but always with swelling) suggests infection, crystal arthritis, or spontaneous haemarthrosis.
- In the very elderly, traumatic lesions may be missed, as presentation is not always so striking, e.g. intra-articular fracture with haemarthrosis.
- An insidious onset of pain is usual in cleavage tears of menisci (horizontal tears), which occur typically in adults where the disc is degenerate, in adolescents with discoid menisci and in early ostochondritis dissecans.

Ask about the pattern and type of pain

- Pain from synovitis is often associated with stiffness and is often worse after a period of immobility. Almost without exception knee synovitis can occur in all forms of arthritis.
- Pain from subchondral damage is almost always worse on weight-bearing, e.g. OA, but this association is not specific.
- Pain on kneeling/squatting is characteristic of anterior knee pain.
- Burning pain may be neurogenic, e.g. L3 nerve root or algodystrophy pain.
- Florid descriptors of pain are often used in algodystrophy.

Past medical, family, occupational, and leisure history

- Knee synovitis and patellar enthesitis occur in adult and juvenile enthesitis-related arthritis. Ask about previous uveitis, low back pain, urethral discharge, sexually transmitted disease, dysentery, and psoriasis.
- Gout is not uncommon around the knee. Ask about gout risk factors and whether the patient has ever had first MTPJ pain (70% of gout sufferers).
- There may be a family history of generalized OA, a hereditary disease of connective tissue or hypermobility in young adults with OA.
- Prepatellar bursitis classically occurred in housemaids! Friction caused by repeated kneeling (occupational) can cause it.
- Sports injuries are common. Anterior cruciate injury occurs characteristically in rugby. Meniscal injuries are common in soccer. Jumping events (e.g. high jump, basketball) can lead to patellar tendon apophysitis. Cycling is associated with anterior knee pain. MCL and meniscal injuries are common in skiing and weight-bearing activities where rotation and change of direction are frequent. Cycling and running are associated with ITB/bursa pain and inflammation.

Examination

From front and behind, observe the patient standing

- Look for mechanical abnormalities that might be associated with knee lesions: patella asymmetry, prominent tibial tubercles from previous Osgood–Schlatter's (anterior knee pain), flat feet, and hypermobility (patella dislocation, hyperextension of >10°).

- Check for mechanical abnormalities which might suggest specific pathology: genu varum (bowed leg, typical appearance with primarily medial compartment OA), obvious suprapatellar knee swelling (synovitis), psoriasis (associated synovitis or enthesitis).
- Marked genu varum occurs in the rare Blount's disease (developmental abnormality of the medial tibial physis typically in Afro-Caribbean boys).

Examination of the sitting patient

Ask the patient to sit on the couch with legs hanging, knees bent. Patellar tracking and pain from medial meniscus damage can be assessed. An alternative approach is with the patient supine. Observe any muscle wasting. Palpate anterior, medial, and lateral structures.

- In patients with anterior knee pain look for symmetrical patellar alignment.
- Observe active knee extension. Patellar movement should be smooth, pain-free, and symmetrical.
- Passively externally rotate each lower leg to its extreme. This is a reasonably sensitive test for conditions of the medial knee compartment (e.g. meniscus tear) and medial knee structures. Discomfort will be felt. If the MCL is totally deficient an abnormally increased range of external rotation may occur.
- Quadriceps wasting (accentuated depression in muscle just above the patella) occurs with disuse after injuries and in chronic arthropathies.
- Sites of bursae, patellar tendon, and ligament insertions should be palpated in patients with localized pain (see Fig. 2.16).
- Tibiofemoral joint line tenderness is likely to be due to either meniscus pathology or marginal osteophytes. Osteophytes give bony swelling.
- Anterior pain from patellofemoral joint disorders may be elicited by gentle pressure down on the patella. Mobilizing the patella sideways will give an impression of tissue laxity (possible underlying hypermobility).
- Factors that predispose to patellofemoral pain syndrome include: high or lateral patella, weak vastus medialis, excessive pronation, weak ankle dorsiflexors, tight hamstrings, reduced movement at the ankle, and a wide Q-angle. The Q-angle is formed between a line from the anterior superior iliac spine to the centre of the patella, and a line extended upwards from the tibial tubercle through the centre of the patella. The larger the angle the greater the lateral tensile pull on the patella (see Fig. 2.15).
- Localized tenderness of the femoral condyle is often the only sign of osteochondritis dissecans in adolescents. The commonest site is on the inside of the medial femoral condyle (75%).

Examine for joint synovitis (synovial inflammation giving synovial thickening and/or tenderness) and an effusion

- The joint may be warm. Chronic synovitis does not always result in a warm joint but infection, crystal arthritis, and haemarthrosis usually do.
- Gross synovitis can produce obvious effusions and/or synovial thickening most easily felt around the patellar edges.
- Effusions may be confirmed by the patellar tap test.

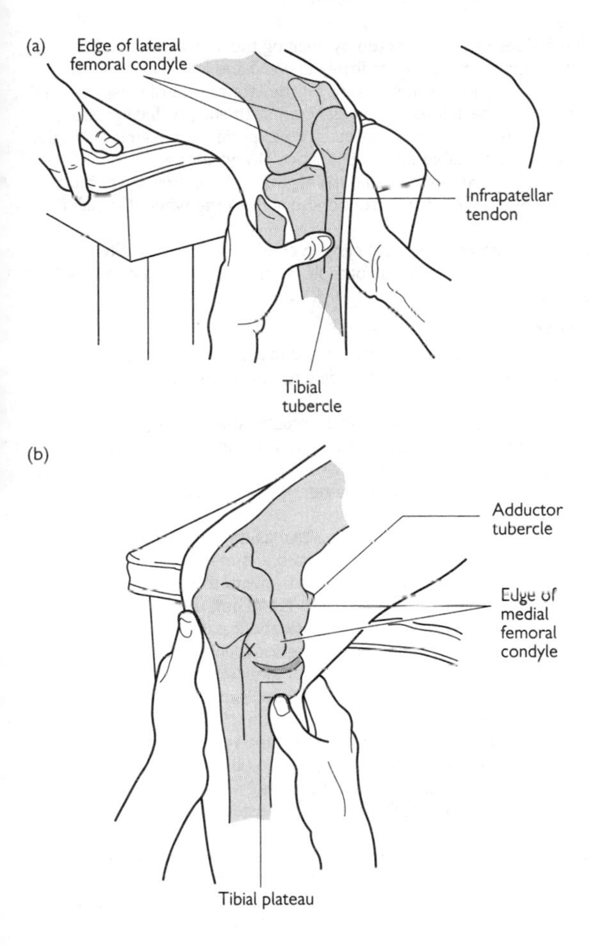

Fig. 2.16 Position of the knee for palpation of most of its structures. Palpating for enthesitis at the patellar tendon insertion (a) Palpation over the insertion of semimembranosus and pes anserinus under the tibial plateau (b) The site of the majority of osteochondritis lesions in the knee is shown by the 'X'

- Small effusions can be detected by eliciting the 'bulge sign'. Fluid in the medial compartment is swept firmly upward and laterally into the suprapatellar pouch. Firm pressure on the lateral side of the joint may then push fluid back into the medial compartment producing a bulge.
- Thickened synovium can be detected by experienced examiners in the absence of a detectable effusion. It is not always tender.
- Posterior compartment synovial thickening and popliteal cysts can be felt by wrapping the fingers around under the knee when it is slightly flexed.
- In contrast to adults, popliteal cysts in children are not usually associated with intra-articular pathology. Investigation is not always necessary.

Test the knee for stability

- There are many tests for instability: instability may be straight or rotatory and can be graded according to consensus criteria (consult orthopaedics texts).
- The Lachmann test (see Fig. 2.17) is arguably the most sensitive test for eliciting anterior cruciate disruption: hold the knee flexed between 20–30°, grasped above and below the joint. Attempt to move the tibia forwards and backwards on the femur. Ask about pain and feel for laxity or a 'clunk'.
- The anterior draw test is not as sensitive as the Lachmann test for detecting partial anterior cruciate tears but is easier to do. The patient lies flat, hip flexed, the knee flexed at 90°, with the foot flat on the couch. Fix the foot by gently sitting on it and pull the top of the lower leg forwards in the line of the thigh. Ask about pain and feel for laxity.
- The posterior draw test identifies posterior cruciate disruption: with the knee flexed to 90°, press the top of the lower leg backwards in the line of the thigh, ask about pain and feel for laxity.
- Test medial stability at 0° and 30° of flexion (MCL stabilizes maximally at 30°) by holding the upper leg still and applying a valgus force to the tibia. Laxity associated with widening of the tibiofemoral joint (with or without pain) is a positive test and suggests MCL deficiency.
- Lateral (LCL and ITB) stability is similarly tested, though using a varus force on the lower leg.
- MCL tears can accompany anterior cruciate injuries and deep lesions are associated with simultaneous tears of the medial meniscus. Such complex pathology can make specific examination manoeuvres difficult to interpret.

Test for meniscus damage

- McMurray's test (see Fig. 2.18). Flex the knee, internally rotate the lower leg, then extend the joint. Repeat with the lower leg externally rotated. The fingers (over the joint line) may feel a 'clunk' as a femoral condyle passes over a torn meniscus. It is often +ve (21–65% of cases) when surgery subsequently reveals no tear.
- Ask the patient to turn over. Lying initially on their side allows you to do Ober's test to detect lateral soft tissue injury. When prone, look and palpate for swelling in the popliteal fossa and proximal calf (low lying popliteal cyst).

Anterior draw test

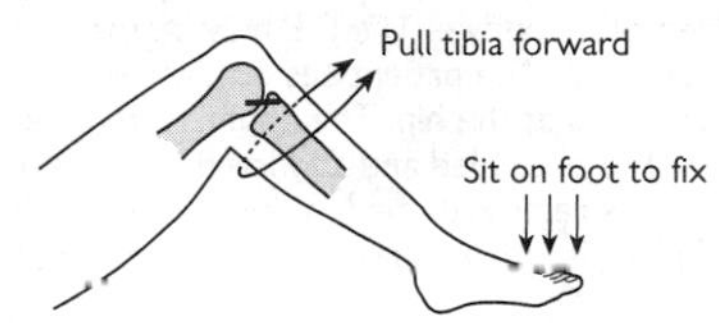

Lachmann test

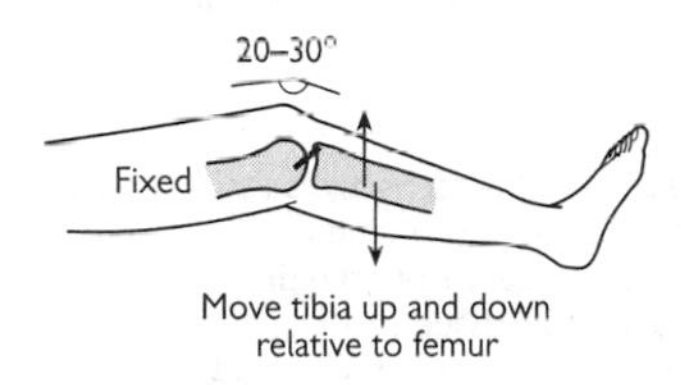

Fig. 2.17 Dynamic tests of anterior cruciate function. Patients should be relaxed lying supine on a couch. Excessive laxity is the most important sign

McMurray's test

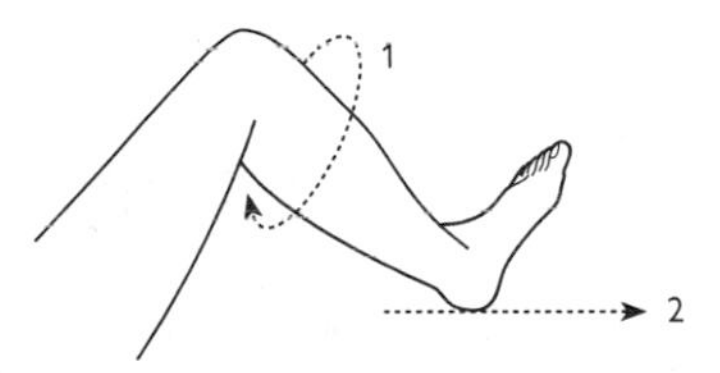

Action: Hold the knee and the heel.
Internally rotate the lower leg (1) then extend it (2)

Positive test: (Palpable) clunk at joint line

Fig. 2.18 Dynamic test designed to elicit signs of meniscus damage. 'Clunks', intra-articular pain, and coarse crepitus may indicate damage. The test is not specific and is open to misinterpretation

- Inflammation of the bursa underlying the ITB may result in tenderness over the lateral femoral condyle. The ITB may be tight. This is demonstrated using Ober's test. The patient lies on their side with the lower (non-affected) leg flexed at the hip. The upper (painful) knee is flexed to 90° and the thigh is extended and adducted. The test is +ve if, when the examiner's hand is removed, the hip does not drop down (further stretching the ITB). Leg length inequality and foot over-pronation may be causative factors.
- Detecting specific structures in the posterior fossa is often difficult because of the lack of bony landmarks and overlapping soft tissue structures. Synovial cysts may form under pressure and are often hard and tender. Diffuse thickening suggests joint synovitis.

Investigations

Radiographs

AP and lateral weight-bearing radiographs are suitable screening views if the diagnosis is unclear after clinical assessment.

- Early synovitis may only be evident from the presence of an effusion, periarticular osteopenia, or soft tissue swelling. Patterns of bone damage in chronic arthropathies may be recognized.
- Signs of joint infection, which may not necessarily present acutely, are patchy bone osteolysis and irregular loss of bone cortex. Osteonecrosis is uncommon in the knee although it occurs in sickle cell anaemia.
- Loss of joint space, angulation deformity, osteophytes, subchondral bone sclerosis, and bone cysts are hallmark features of OA.
- In adults, linear or vague intra-articular calcification suggests chondrocalcinosis (associated with calcium pyrophosphate dihydrate (CPPD) arthritis). Gross 'thumbprint' calcification is typical of synovial chondromatosis (mainly in children).
- In children check for an osteochondral fragment (e.g. osteochondritis dissecans), normal epiphyses, epiphyseal plates and metaphyses, normal patella shape, and osteochondritis at the tibial tubercle (see Table 2.21).

Specialized radiographic views: tomographic views; 'skyline' (axial with knee bent) view; or lateral view taken with at least 30° of flexion

- Tomography is useful for clarifying non-peripheral osteochondral defects.
- Skyline views demonstrate anomalous patellar facet configuration and can reveal patellofemoral incongruity though multiple views may be needed. Subchondral patellar pathology is seen more clearly than on lateral views.
- Patella alta is most reliably seen on a lateral view with 30° flexion.

Further imaging

Further imaging depends on differential diagnosis and a discussion with your radiologist:

- Periarticular soft tissue lesions can be characterized with MR, though with superficial lesions adequate information needed for further management may be obtainable with ultrasound alone.

Table 2.21 Interpretation of radiographic knee abnormalities in children

Radiographic abnormality	Possible conditions (most commonly)
Intra-articular calcific fragment	Osteochondritis dissecans, traumatic avulsion, synovial tumours, or chondromatosis (rare)
Epiphyseal defect/abnormality	JIA, sepsis, avulsion injury, bone dysplasias, rickets, haemophilia, hypothyroidism
Transverse radiolucent metaphyseal band or lysis	Leukaemia, lymphoma, neuroblastoma metastases, infections (neonates), osteogenesis imperfecta, idiopathic juvenile osteoporosis, Cushing's disease
Joint space narrowing	JIA, sepsis, PVNS, haemophilia
Diffuse low bone density	Rickets, OI, osteoporosis, mucopolysaccharidosis
Periosteal reaction	Fracture, sepsis, infarction, tumours matosis (rare)

- Patterns of meniscus damage are recognized on MR, give an indication of prognosis, and aid the surgeon's decision to proceed to arthroscopy.
- MR is essential if there is likely to be a combination of lesions, e.g. anterior cruciate, MCL, and medial meniscus lesions.
- In children, both US and MR will confirm synovitis.
- MR is more sensitive in identifying joint erosions in RA compared than are radiographs or US.
- The place of CT or MR in investigating radiographically detected bone tumours depends on the likely nature of the lesion.

Aspiration of joint and periarticular fluid collections

⚠ Early aspiration is essential if infection is suspected.

- The knee is a common site of monoarthritis. The principles behind management apply to all cases of single joint pathology.
- Send joint fluid for microscopy and culture of gonococcus in adolescents and young adults, and TB as well as routine bacterial pathogens.
- In adults, the usual differential diagnosis of sepsis of knee structures is gout, so fluid should be examined by polarized light microscopy for urate crystals.
- Blood-stained fluid either suggests a traumatic tap or chondrocalcinosis. Frank blood suggests haemarthrosis, the major causes of which are cruciate tear, bleeding diathesis, intra-articular fracture, and pigmented villonodular synovitis (PVNS).
- Bursa fluid may be more successfully detected and aspirated using US guidance.

Laboratory investigations

These should be directed towards suspected underlying disease:

- FBC/CBC, acute phase response (ESR, CRP).
- Blood urea, electrolytes, creatinine, and urate.
- Blood calcium, phosphate, albumin, ALP, 25-OH vit D (± PTH) to screen for metabolic bone disease.
- Autoantibodies: rheumatoid factor (RF), antinuclear (ANA), and extractable nuclear antibodies (ENAs) to characterize an autoimmune process where synovitis is chronic.
- Serum angiotensin converting enzyme (sACE) for sarcoid.
- IgM *Borrelia burgdorferi* serology for acute arthropathy in Lyme disease, streptococcal antibodies for reactive strep. arthritis.

Treatment

- In general most soft tissue lesions will settle with rest and NSAIDs.
- Anterior knee pain may respond well to isometric exercises, adjustments to foot alignment, e.g. sensible shoes and foot orthoses (support insoles) and hamstring stretching exercises.
- The acute swollen knee requires aspiration, rest for 24 h and gentle mobilization. If infection is considered, broad-spectrum antibiotics against staphylococcal and streptococcal agents should be started immediately pending results of cultures. In infection, intra-articular antibiotics and steroids should be avoided. The patient should not bear weight on an acutely infected joint.
- Acute and chronic inflammation can lead to joint destruction and instability. If RA, treat early.
- Physiotherapy and splinting play an important role in maintaining function and preventing contractures etc.

Address biomechanical factors

Physiotherapy input may be helpful in cases of anterior knee pain. Success from McConnell (patellar) taping is more likely in nonpatellofemoral OA-related anterior knee pain.

- Quadriceps strengthening exercises can be reviewed and reinforced by physiotherapists in cases of knee OA.
- Knee pain, particularly anterior pain, may be linked to foot abnormalities, e.g. overpronation, and hip alignment (see Q-angle, above). Specific muscle strengthening exercises, foot orthotics, and knee braces should be considered.

Local steroid injection

Local steroid injections can be helpful in the following situations:

- Acute flare of non-infective inflammatory disease:
  - OA (especially where CPPD is present—mild OA may also respond to hyaluronate injections
  - autoimmune arthritis, e.g. RA, SpA
  - intra-articular gout
  - SpA, etc.
- Bursitis (may be gout):
  - pre- and infrapatella (superficial and deep) bursa (the latter may require US guidance)
  - anserine.

- Baker's cyst (note: the knee joint is injected at the site of the 1° pathology assuming there is intra-articular communication between joint and cyst. Direct popliteal cyst injection should be under US guidance only).
- Enthesopathy, e.g. semimembranosus insertion.
- Trauma, e.g. pain over medial collateral ligament insertion.
- Other soft-tissue: ITB syndrome.

The reader is referred to p.148 for steroid injection techniques and to part 2 chapters for specific diseases.

Joint injection therapies

- Needle arthrocentesis with saline irrigation may be helpful in treating knee OA.
- Radiation synovectomy using yttrium-90 (Y-90) colloid or dysprosium-165 ferric hydroxymacroaggregates given before there is evidence of advanced chondral loss are useful adjuncts in managing inflammatory arthritis. Long-acting steroid should be co-injected.
- Y-90 has been shown to be effective in CPPD and, in uncontrolled series, in haemophilic arthritis.
- There is anecdotal evidence for the efficacy of intra-articular osmic acid injection (chemical synonectomy) in inflammatory arthritis. It may be preferred to Y-90 in juvenile idiopathic arthritis given the risks of using radiation in children.

Note; all intra-articular injection therapies are more effective when patients' knees are immobilized (bed rest or strong splint) for 48 h following the procedure.

Drugs

- NSAIDs will invariably be helpful in cases of inflammatory and infective arthritis.
- Colchicine 0.5 mg up to 2–3-hourly is often useful in relieving pain from crystal arthritis in patients intolerant of NSAIDs.
- In randomized trials, paracetamol is as effective as NSAIDs.
- Glucosamine has been shown to have an analgesic effect and improves function in OA. It may slow the rate of cartilage loss.

See part 2 chapters for specific treatment of chronic autoimmune arthritides.

Surgery

- Arthroscopy is often used as a diagnostic tool in cases of undiagnosed monoarthritis and to confirm and trim cartilage tears. Synovium and synovial lesions (e.g. PVNS, synovial chondromatosis) can be biopsied or excised (synovectomy) and the joint can be irrigated.
- In appropriate cases joint replacement can be remarkably successful and is an important option to consider in OA and inflammatory arthritis where pain is severe and present at rest, and when mobility is substantially restricted.
- Arthrodesis is rarely indicated.
- Unicondylar osteotomy can aid realignment of the tibiofemoral joint, e.g. in metabolic bone disease such as Paget's disease.

Other

- In OA, capsaicin cream applied three or four times daily to painful superficial structures, e.g. patellar margins or marginal tibiofemoral joint pain, can ease symptoms. Response may not occur for 6–8 weeks.
- There is anecdotal evidence for external beam radiotherapy in treating inflammatory lesions, e.g. enthesitis. In appropriate patients the relative risks are negligible (e.g. the elderly and those at high risk from systemic medications).

Lower leg and foot disorders (adults)

Anatomy

Anatomy of bones and joints

- The leg absorbs six times the body weight during weight-bearing. Strong ligaments secure the ankle (formed by tibia above/medially and fibular malleolus laterally) and talocalcaneal (subtalar) joints and bones of the midfoot (see Fig. 2.19).
- Anomalous ossicles in the foot are common. Some are associated with specific pathology. There are many potential sites, though the sesamoids in flexor hallucis brevis (FHB) are invariable.
- The foot is an optimal mechanical device to support body weight when walking or running over flat, inclined, and uneven types of terrain. The configuration of, and synchronous movements between, bones at synovial articulations allows dorsal flexion (foot pulled up), plantar flexion (to walk on toes), inversion (foot tips in), eversion (foot tips out), and small degrees of adduction and abduction. Midfoot movements allow pronation and supination.
- The normal ankle joint range is about 25° of dorsal flexion and 50° of plantar flexion from neutral (foot 90° to leg). The range of subtalar inversion–eversion is normally 10–15°.

Anatomy of the long muscles and tendons

- In the lower leg a strong fascia connects the tibia and fibula. Lower leg muscles primarily move the foot. They are separated into compartments by fasciae and are prone to pressure effects.
- The foot dorsal flexors—tibialis anterior, extensor digitorum longus (EDL), extensor hallucis longus (EHL) and peroneus tertius—lie adjacent to the anteromedial side of the tibia. Their tendons pass in front of the ankle in synovial sheaths held down by strong retinaculae (see Fig. 2.20). Tibialis anterior, the bulkiest, inserts into the medial midfoot (medial cuneiform).
- In the posterior lower leg gastrocnemius (and plantaris), which arises from the femur, plantar flexes the foot by levering up the back of the calcaneum. Soleus, which arises in the lower leg, merges with them in the Achilles' tendon. The tendon has a deep and superficial bursa at its insertion site.
- Plantar flexion is assisted weakly by long muscles, which arise in the lower leg, pass behind the medial malleolus in synovial sheaths (see Fig. 2.20), and insert into the sole. They mostly invert the foot. Tibialis posterior, the most bulky, inserts into the plantar surface of the navicular.
- Peroneus longus and brevis arise from the fibular side of the leg and pass around the lateral malleolus in a common synovial sheath held by a retinaculum. Longus passes into the sole and inserts into the medial cuneiform. Brevis inserts into the fifth metatarsal base. Both evert the foot.
- The tibial nerve and artery follow the course of the medial tendons under the flexor retinaculum (see Fig. 2.20).

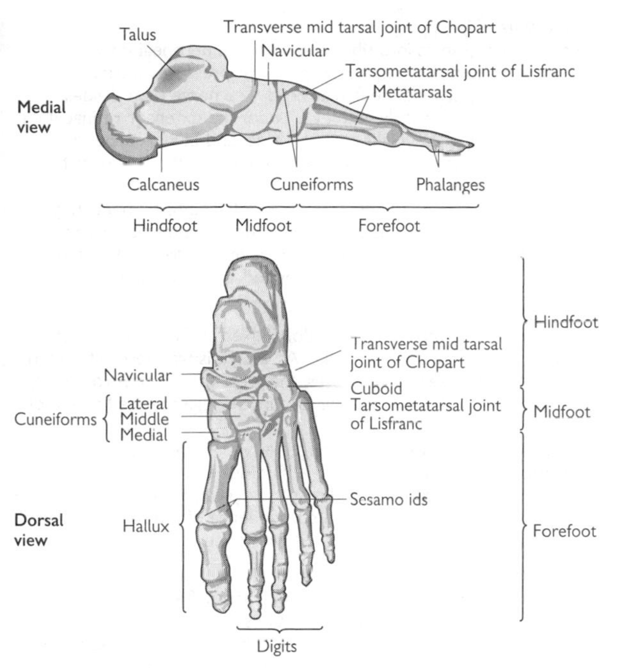

Fig. 2.19 The bones of the foot

Anatomy of intrinsic foot structure

- Intrinsic foot structures have been greatly modified during evolution to combine provision of a sprung platform for support and a rigid lever for thrusting body weight forward when walking.
- In the sole of the foot, muscles are aligned longitudinally in four layers. The deepest layers include phalangeal interossei in the forefeet, tibialis posterior, peroneus longus, adductor hallucis, and FHB—which has two insertions into the proximal great toe phalanx, each containing a sesamoid.
- The superficial layers include flexor digitorum longus (FDL), which inserts into the lateral four distal phalanges, the phalangeal lumbricals, flexor digitorum brevis, and abductor hallucis. The latter two muscles arise from the plantar surface of the calcaneum deep to the plantar fascia.
- Flexor tendons merge with the deeper part of the plantar fascia, a swath of tissue that extends from os calcis to the metatarsal area.
- Longitudinal muscles, ligaments, and fascia contribute to stabilize the foot with a longitudinal arch—its apex at the talus but also with some effect laterally. The foot arches transversely—its apex at medial cuneiform level.

Neuroanatomy

- The sciatic nerve splits into tibial and common peroneal nerves above the knee. The common peroneal is prone to pressure neuropathy as it runs superficially around the fibular head. The nerve then divides. A deep branch runs distally with EDL under the extensor retinaculum to the foot. It supplies tibialis anterior, EHL, and EDL. A superficial branch supplies the peroneal muscles and most of the skin over the dorsum of the foot.
- The tibial nerve runs in the posterior lower leg compartment supplying gastrocnemius and soleus. It then passes under the medial flexor retinaculum dividing into medial and lateral plantar nerves, which supply the intrinsic plantar muscles of the foot and skin of the sole.

Functional anatomy

- In a normal gait pattern the foot is dorsiflexed and invertors/evertors stabilize the hindfoot for heel strike. As weight is transferred forwards the foot plantar flexes and pronates, the great toe extends (optimally between 65 and 75°), and push off occurs through the medial side of the forefoot.
- All metatarsals bear weight and can suffer weight-bearing injury.
- Ligamentous attachments around the hindfoot are strong. A fall on a pronated inverted foot without direct trauma can result in a fracture of the distal fibula. This is probably a consequence of the relative strength of the talofibular ligaments compared with bone.

Developmental factors

- Developmental characteristics often imply that different age groups are prone to a different spectrum of conditions.
- Due to ligamentous laxity, when babies begin to walk the midfoot is flat to the floor. A longitudinal arch usually develops by 5 years.
- During growth, tendon insertions (apophyses) are often weaker than the tendons themselves. Traction strain on tendons can lead to apophysitis (osteochondritis). This is a common pattern of injury in the foot in active older children.

Conditions of the lower leg

- Patients with lower leg conditions may present with pain or deformity alone. In children, deformity may typically be due to spinal dysraphism (from birth), rickets (acquired age 1 year plus), or osteogenesis imperfecta.
- Pains in the calf may be due to local soft tissue or muscle conditions but in adults are commonly due to referred lumbosacral pain. These pains are often described by patients as 'cramps'—suggesting a muscle problem at first. A detailed history may suggest nerve root pathology.

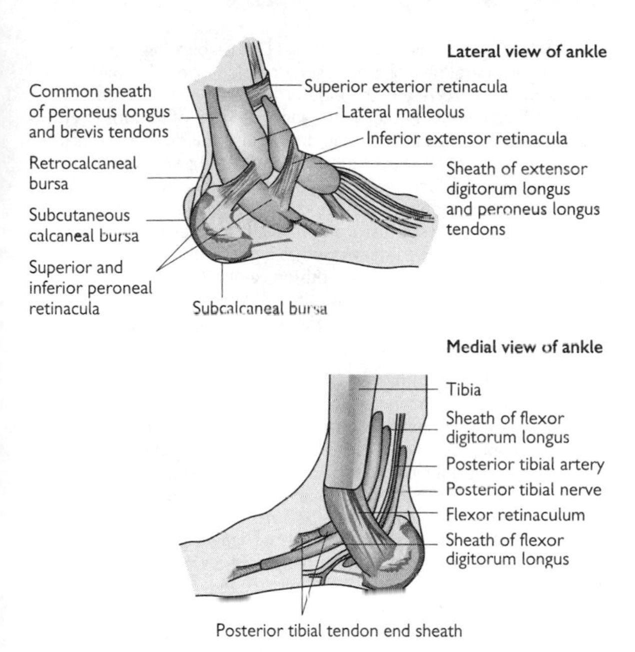

Fig. 2.20 Tendons, retinaculae, and bursae of the hindfoot

- Imbalance of muscles in the foot can lead to ↑ tension at tendon and fascial insertions in the calf and shin, resulting in 'shin splints'. Shin splints usually present after activity and are relieved by rest. Conditions to consider include:
  - stress fractures of the tibia of fibula
  - tibialis posterior fasciitis—often associated with a flat, pronated foot
  - compartment syndrome (soft tissue and vascular swelling)
  - popliteal artery stenosis
  - referred nerve pain (spinal claudication)
  - peripheral vascular disease (intermittent claudication).

Taking a history

Ask about site and quality of pain in the lower leg

- Localized anterior pain occurs in bony lesions of the anterior tibia, e.g. stress fractures, periositis etc. (see 'shin splints' above).

- Burning pain suggests a neurogenic cause. Diffuse burning pain may be caused by peripheral neuropathy, algodystrophy, or erythromelalgia.
- Most commonly occurring in the elderly, bilateral leg pain with 'heaviness' or 'stiffness' limiting walking distance is typical of lumbosacral canal stenosis. An alternative would be vascular claudication where often pain is more overt, and critical ischaemia can give night pain eased by hanging the legs over the side of the bed (gravity effects).
- Simultaneous knee problems may be relevant. Escape of synovial fluid from the knee into the soft tissues of the calf can present with acute pain and swelling and be misdiagnosed as a deep vein thrombosis. Often a history of preceding joint effusion can be elicited.
- Low-lying synovial cysts connecting with the knee can cause calf pain (with or without swelling). This invariably occurs only with chronic synovitis.

Establish possible causes of hindfoot pain (Table 2.22)

- Establishing the cause of hindfoot pain from the history alone is difficult. There are important clues, mainly from patterns of injury/overuse.
- Posterior heel pain has a few causes. Often clinically indistinguishable from Achilles tendonitis or retrocalcaneal bursitis, enthesitis is usually associated with SpA. An os trigonum may become damaged especially in soccer players and ballerinas (see below).
- The origin of plantar heel pain is varied. Mechanical plantar fasciitis is thought to occur more frequently in people who are on their feet for long periods of time, those who are obese, have thin heel fat pads, or poor footwear. Symptoms of arthritis and enthesopathy elsewhere, low back pain (sacroiliitis), eye inflammation (iritis), psoriasis, or previous gut or 'urethral' infection, might suggest a link of 1° inflammatory plantar fasciitis with SpA.
- Less common causes of plantar heel pain include fracture through a calcaneal spur and lateral plantar nerve entrapment between the fascia of abductor hallucis and quadratus plantae muscles (causing pain/parasthesiae on the lateral side of the sole).
- In the elderly and postmenopausal women calcaneal stress fractures are a recognized feature of osteoporosis and can present with heel pain.
- Ankle and talocalcaneal synovitis, OA, ankle osteochondritis dissecans, and tendonitis around the hindfoot may be difficult to distinguish from the history alone. Synovitis or an effusion often accompanies OA of these joints.

Establish possible causes of midfoot and first MTP pain

- Gout, OA, enthesitis, and referred L5 nerve root pain are the likeliest diagnoses of midfoot and first MTP pain.
- Any joint may potentially become involved in the major chronic arthropathies.

Table 2.22 Common conditions causing localized foot pain in children, adolescents, and adults

Site of pain	Common lesions
Ankle region	Ankle or talocalcaneal joint: synovitis (e.g. gout), OA. L4/L5 root pain
Posterior heel	Achilles tendonitis. Retrocalcaneal bursitis. Achilles enthesitis. Osteonecrosis of os trigonum
Medial side of heel	As for ankle region. Calcaneal fracture. Tibialis posterior tendonitis. Plantar fasciitis.
Lateral side of heel	As for ankle region. Calcaneal fracture. Peroneal tendonitis. Fifth metatarsal base fracture*
Underneath heel	Plantar fasciitis. Calcaneal fracture. Infracalcaneal bursitis. Lateral plantar nerve entrapment
Top of foot	Midfoot joint synovitis (e.g. gout), OA. Navicular osteochondritis. Enthesitis. L5 root pain
Sole of foot	S1 root pain. Plantar fasciitis. Metatarsal stress fracture. Tibial/plantar nerve entrapment
Toes	MTPJ synovitis (e.g. RA, gout). MTPJ OA. Morton's metatarsalgia. Bursitis. Enthesitis/dactylitis

*Robert–Jones fracture from an inversion–pronation injury.

- Gout should always be considered a possible cause of painful lesions in the foot in people at risk. Gout is not always intra-articular, intrabursal, or intratendonal. Local or diffuse soft tissue inflammation is common and often misdiagnosed as cellulitis. Swelling is usually marked.
- L5 pain is referred to the top (dorsum) and S1 pain to the sole of the foot.
- In older adults OA of midfoot joints is common. Mild synovitis can occur with it and may be caused by CPPD crystals.

Establish possible causes of forefoot pain

- In those with forefoot pain, typically referred to as metatarsalgia, establish whether the condition is focal or due to arthropathy.
- Pain under the ball of the foot whilst walking is non-specific but might suggest any MTPJ abnormality, distal metatarsal stress fracture, Freiberg's disease, planter nerve neuroma, or bursitis.
- Patients with RA often describe pain under the MTPJs and a feeling of 'walking on pebbles' (due to joint swelling and/or subluxation). Synovitis of the MTPJs is a very common feature of early RA.
- Acute pain under the forefoot spreading into one or more (adjacent) toes and worse on walking suggests a plantar nerve neuroma (Morton's metatarsalgia) or intermetatarsal bursitis.
- Pain associated with parasthesiae or numbness under the forefoot might be due to S1 root irritation (common) or entrapment of the tibial nerve in the hindfoot (rare). Ask about back pain and other hindfoot problems.

- Non-traumatic toe pain associated with entire toe swelling suggests a dactylitis (associated with SpA). Although many toes may be affected, the dactylitis may be unilateral and affect just one toe.
- The development of hallux valgus is associated with tight footwear. The established deformity is associated with altered weight-bearing and a second toe (hammer) deformity. Big toe pain might be due to hallux rigidus. It is usually 2° to OA and important to recognize as it may prevent toe dorsiflexion sufficiently to lead to a compromized gait pattern.
- Pain specifically under the hallux may be due to damage of the sesamoids in the flexor hallucis brevis tendon and be misdiagnosed as a joint problem.

Ask for a description of the pain

- As in the hand, neurogenic pain is common and typical.
- Severe or unremitting pain when at rest suggests intrinsic bone pathology. Consider osteonecrosis, infection, fracture, and tumours, e.g. osteoid osteoma.
- Neurogenic pain may be sharp and well-defined (e.g. in acute L5 or S1 root pain, (see p.82)), deep, achy, and less well-defined (e.g. chronic nerve root symptoms as in spinal or foramenal stenosis) or burning in quality. Parasthesiae and numbness may accompany both.
- If swelling accompanies neurogenic pain, consider algodystrophy. There are numerous triggers, e.g. trauma, surgery. Patients may be unwilling to walk and apparent disability may appear profound.

Weakness (?)

If true weakness is the major problem rather than pain, the diagnosis is usually between a spinal and peripheral nerve lesion (see Examination, below).

Examination

Observation

Observe the lower legs and feet from front and back whilst the patient is standing. Note any swelling, deformities, or rashes:

- Lower leg deformities to note: tibia varum (or bow legs) in an older adult may be due to Paget's disease of the tibia. Muscle wasting might suggest disuse atrophy, old polio, or lumbosacral spinal canal stenosis (bilateral and subtle usually in older adults).
- Oedema or soft tissue swelling may be relevant to an underlying condition, e.g. RA. Although it may cause discomfort, oedema from cardiac failure, venous congestion, and hypoproteinaemia and lymphoedema is not painful unless there are ulcers or thrombophlebitis.
- Gout can cause swelling anywhere.
- Calf swelling may be due to vein thrombosis or ruptured popliteal cyst.
- Common patterns of foot deformity are:
  - flat feet (pes planus)
  - high-arched feet (pes cavus) with high medial arch
  - hallux valgus and rigidus
  - overriding, hammer, and claw toes.
- Skin conditions from venous abnormalities are common in the elderly. Other skin lesions which may be relevant include purpura, panniculitis—which is often subtle and over the shins—and pyoderma gangrenosum.

Ask the patient to walk in bare feet

Gait patterns should be noted:

- An antalgic ('limp and wince') gait is a non-specific indicator of pain.
- A wide-based gait (>10 cm wider than normal) suggests instability: joint instability, muscle weakness, or neurological lesions may be the cause.
- A foot that slaps down or a high stepping gait suggests tibialis anterior weakness (L4 nerve root or common peroneal nerve lesion).
- Significant weakness of gluteus medius and gluteus maximus in L5 and S1 root lesions respectively can result in lurching during gait. In the former, as weight is taken on the affected side, gluteus medius may be weak in controlling the small 2–3 cm lateral displacement in the weight-bearing hip that normally occurs. This can be compensated for if the body centre of gravity is brought over the hip by lurching the upper body over the affected side. With gluteus maximus lesions (S1) extension of the hip, which helps mediate motion through the stance phase prior to toeing-off, may be weak. Thrusting the thorax forward with an arched back (forward lurch) compensates for the weakness and helps to maintain hip extension.
- A flat-footed gait with little or weak toe-off may suggest an S1 root lesion; however, 'flat-foot' (loss of the medial arch) with associated hind foot eversion and heel pain (plantar fasciitis) is extremely common. Often the arch weakness corrects when the patient is asked to walk.

Examine the lower leg

With the patient supine on the couch, examine the lower leg:

- After a ruptured popliteal cyst, calf tissues are often diffusely tender and swollen. Calf circumferences can be compared (e.g. 10 cm below tibial tubercle). There may also be mild skin erythema. Findings are not specific. Gout and infection are the main alternatives if there is marked tenderness. A DVT causes relatively painless swelling.
- Check for bruising, swelling, and tenderness around the fibula head in patients with foot drop (possible peroneal nerve palsy). Neurological examination may be done at this point.
- Localized anterior tibial tenderness is often found in patients with stress fractures or with pseudofractures (osteomalacia).
- Tibial deformity in adults may be associated with diffuse bony tenderness and heat (arteriovenous shunting) in Paget's disease.

Examine the ankle and hindfoot

At the ankle and hindfoot, examine for joint and tendon synovitis, palpate specific structures and test passive hindfoot joint mobility:

- Synovitis of hindfoot joints is not always easily detected. With ankle joint synovitis, thickened tissue may be felt anteriorly in the ankle crease (where there may be a 'springy fullness') or laterally around the malleoli.

- Posterior tibial and peroneal tendonitis are associated with soft tissue swelling of the medial and lateral hindfoot respectively. Synovial thickening from ankle and talocalcaneal joints may also be felt here and synovitis of structures may coexist in RA or SpA. Pain from resisted movement of tendons may not be specific.
- Pathology of medial hindfoot structures may be associated with tibial nerve entrapment resulting in sensory symptoms on the sole of the foot. There may be a positive Tinnel's sign.
- Posterior heel pain may be due to Achilles' tendonitis, enthesitis and mechanical damage to the tendon, and retrocalcaneal bursitis. Deep tenderness may suggest an os trigonum lesion.
- The loss of passive hindfoot movements is not specific and can be associated with any cause of ankle or subtalar arthritis (20–30° of dorsiflexion and 45–55° of plantar flexion is average for the ankle and a 10–20° inversion–eversion range is average for the subtalar joint). Subtalar joint movement can be difficult to test accurately.
- The pain of plantar fasciitis may be elicited by firm palpation of the medial underside of the calcaneum. A negative test does not rule out pathology, as often the history is more sensitive. Full musculoskeletal examination is required to check for features of SpA such as arthritis/enthesitis elsewhere and sacroiliitis.

Examine for midfoot lesions

Identifying specific midfoot lesions is difficult, though bony landmarks and discrete tender areas can be noted:

- Twisting the midfoot may elicit pain non-specifically. Common lesions include gout, OA, and synovitis associated with RA and SpA.
- Bony tenderness alone without soft tissue swelling does not rule out synovitis of an adjacent joint.
- The midfoot is a typical site for neuroarthropathy in diabetes.
- Bony lumps (exostoses) that may have formed at sites of pressure are common in the foot (e.g. medial or dorsal aspect of the first MTPJ, base or head of the fifth metatarsal, distal talus, or over the midfoot). In the elderly bony pain and skin sores may form at these sites.
- Both gout and infection result in swelling, skin erythema and localized tenderness. Gout of the first MTPJ occurs at any one time in 70% of patients with the condition. It can occur anywhere in the foot.

Examine the forefoot

Check for bony or other swelling, digit separation, and examine the sole of the foot. Squeezing the whole forefoot at the line of the MTPJs is a non-specific but useful screening test for painful forefoot lesions:

- Tender swelling of the whole toe (dactylitis) occurs in SpA, sarcoid, and HIV infection. Swelling is soft not bony. Tender bony swelling suggests a bunion and is common on the dorsal aspect of the toes and the first and fifth MTPJs.
- Forefoot splaying and interdigital separation suggests MTPJ synovitis or interdigital bursitis. MTPJs may be individually tender (simultaneously palpated with thumb below and finger above).

- Tenderness between metatarsal heads is typical in Morton's metatarsalgia. There may be a sensory deficit in the interdigital cleft. The differential diagnosis (in adolescents) may be osteochondritis of the second and third metatarsal head.
- Check for hallux rigidus—passive dorsiflexion should be at least 50°. Extending the big toe passively can reveal an ability to form a medial longitudinal arch in patients with flat feet (Jack's test).
- Discrete bony tenderness without swelling occurs with stress fractures.
- Uneven callus distribution under the forefoot may suggest an abnormally focused area of weight-bearing and an underlying mechanical abnormality.
- Rashes on the sole of the foot are uncommon but important to consider are: pompholyx, pustular psoriasis, and keratoderma blenhorragica (see Reactive arthritis p.306).
- Loss of sensation under the forefoot may be due to an S1 root lesion, peripheral neuropathy (e.g. diabetes), mononeuritis (e.g. vasculitis, Sjögren's syndrome, mixed connective tissue disease), or, rarely, tibial nerve entrapment (examine hindfoot).

Neurological examination

Neurological examination is essential in cases where pain is neurogenic or there is weakness, numbness, or parasthesiae (see Table 2.23).

Investigations

Imaging of the lower leg

- Suspected tibial abnormalities such as stress fractures and pseudofractures in osteomalacia and Paget's disease have characteristic radiological appearances.
- Periosteal changes occur in trauma, psoriatic arthritis (above ankle), HPOA and pachydermal periostitis
- In athletes with exercise-related pain a three-phase bone scan is part of the work-up for anterior shin pain.
- In suspected (though radiograph-negative) cases of bony disease such as cortical stress fracture, periostitis, or cortical hyperostosis a bone scan is a useful investigation as it is sensitive for these conditions.

Imaging of the foot

Information available on radiographs of the hindfoot includes:

- Increased soft-tissue attenuation around the tendon insertion in cases of Achilles tendonitis or retrocalcaneal bursitis.
- Erosions or periostitis at the Achilles tendon insertion in enthesitis associated with SpA.
- Erosions in gout and RA-associated retrocalcaneal bursitis.
- Axial radiographs of the hindfoot are useful in showing talocalcaneal joint abnormalities, e.g. in RA.
- If radiographs are normal in patients with posterior heel pain, US can show patterns of tendon and bursal inflammation. MR characterizes any discrete pattern of tendon injury further.

Table 2.23 Patterns of common abnormal examination findings in lower lumbar nerve root lesions

Nerve root	Abnormal finding
L4	Weakness of ankle dorsiflexion (tibialis anterior)
	Patient finds walking on their heel difficult (strong ankle dorsiflexion needed)*
	Reduced knee reflex (L3 and L4)
L5	Weakness of big toe dorsiflexion (extensor hallucis longus)
	Weakness of foot eversion (peroneal muscles, also S1)
	Sensory deficit over dorsum of foot
	Reduced ankle reflex (L5 and S1)
S1	Weakness of ankle plantar flexion (gastrocnemius and soleus)
	Patient finds walking on, or repeatedly rising onto, tiptoe difficult*
	Sensory deficit over sole of foot
	Reduced ankle reflex

*Manoeuvres may be affected by pain, making interpretation difficult.

- Osteonecrosis of an os trigonum or posterior talar process or tarsal navicular may be identified by radiographs. It is invariably located by bone scintigraphy and can be characterized further, usually with soft tissue swelling, by MR.
- A plantar spur does not denote current plantar fasciitis.
- Plantar heel pain may be due to a fracture in a spur. Erosions just above the spur may be seen. The thickness of heel fat pad can be gauged from its X-ray attenuation (thin = risk for plantar fasciitis). A fat pad >23 mm thick in men and >21.5 mm thick in women is associated with acromegaly.
- Calcaneal fractures or an osteoid osteoma can be seen in some cases with radiographs alone. Bone scans/CT are more sensitive.
- Patterns of joint, enthesis, and tendon inflammation can be documented using MR but also with a well-executed bone scan. This is useful information when characterizing an arthropathy.
- Bony abnormalities in the mid and forefoot are generally revealed by radiographs alone, though metatarsal stress fractures may be missed. MR can discriminate a plantar neuroma from interdigital bursitis and MTPJ synovitis. The former are probably best initially demonstrated by US.

Other investigations

- Neurophysiology is a useful adjunct to clinical examination in diagnosis of lower limb neuropathies and can help discriminate between peripheral (common peroneal or sciatic) or nerve root causes of foot drop, and also S1 root or tibial nerve entrapment causes of parasthesiae of the sole of the foot.

- Joint/bursa fluid aspiration is mandatory in suspected cases of sepsis and should be sent for culture (remember to consider gonococcus in young adults and TB in patients from endemic or inner-city areas). Fluid should be sent for polarized microscopy if a crystal-induced disease is suspected.
- Laboratory tests requested should reflect suspicion of specific infective, inflammatory, metabolic, or malignant pathology.

Treatment

Lower leg disorders

- Anterior shin pain should be treated according to cause. If there is also a problem of foot alignment then orthoses that support both the hind foot and mid arch may be very useful. Patients may volunteer that good 'training' shoes help (as is the case with plantar fasciitis).
- Exercise-induced lower leg pain has a number of causes and includes shin splints and compartment syndrome. The latter may require further investigation with pressure readings or exercise scintigraphy (^{99m}Tc-MIBI). In cases resistant to rest, analgesia, and modification of triggering factors, decompressive surgery may be required.
- Patients with Paget's disease of the tibia may require treatment with high-dose bisphosphonates and will need a biomechanical assessment.

Ankle and hindfoot disorders

- Tendonitis around the ankle should respond to treatment of its underlying cause. Chronic posterior tibial tendonitis left untreated will eventually accelerate the development of hindfoot valgus. Consider heel and arch support orthotics early.
- Plantar fasciitis may respond to a number of conservative measures:
  - heel pads and/or supportive shoes ('trainers')
  - modification of weight-bearing activity
  - Achilles tendon stretching
  - hindfoot strapping
  - resting night splint (preventing ankle plantar flexion)
  - steroid injection around medial calcaneal tubercle
  - external beam radiotherapy
  - surgery.

Forefoot disorders

- Localized forefoot pain, e.g. metatarsalgia, may respond to support pads and a change to a wider, more supportive, low-heel shoe. A podiatry/chiropody opinion should be sought as required.
- Forefoot stress fractures and metatarsal head osteochondritis require rest, supportive footwear and time to heal.
- Patients with chronic forefoot pain may benefit from a podiatric assessment. 'Stress offloading' foot orthoses for metatarsalgia and other biomechanical abnormalities (e.g. hallux rigidus) can be individually moulded using thermoplastic materials.

Steroid injections (see also p.148)

Steroid injections may be of value in the following:

- Ankle joint inflammation (e.g. RA, OA, gout)
- Subtalar joint inflammation

- Tarsal tunnel syndrome
- Achilles peritendonitis (local steroid injections for Achilles' nodules should be avoided if possible as the risk of rupture is high. The same concern, though probably lesser risk, applies to Achilles' peritendonitis)
- Calcaneal apophysitis (Sever's disease—Achilles' tendon insertion)
- Retrocalcaneal bursitis
- Plantar fasciitis
- Gout/OA/enthesitis at first MTPJ.

Surgery

- Minor surgical techniques can be curative in tarsal tunnel syndrome and in excising an interdigital (Morton's) neuroma. Consider excision of painful exostoses and troublesome rheumatoid nodules and amputation of deformed or over-riding toes.
- Major surgical procedures with good outcomes in appropriate patients include fusion of hindfoot joints and forefoot arthroplasty in chronic inflammatory arthritides. Osteotomy realignment of a hallux valgus deformity can be successful in the long term.

Child and adolescent foot disorders

For a review of classification criteria of autoimmune juvenile arthritides p.193.

Background

Lower limb and foot deformities of babies may be noticed first by parents. Diagnostic evaluation needs to focus on ruling out major congenital disease and exploring biomechanical factors.

- Neonatal deformities of the leg are uncommon.
- Talipes equinovarus (club foot) is an important deformity, which presents at birth. It is most commonly idiopathic and it is associated with wasting of the lower leg muscles. Causes to consider and rule out are spina bifida, spinal dysraphism, cerebral palsy, and arthrogryposis.
- With babies, persistence of certain sleeping postures is associated with patterns of angular and torsion deformity involving the whole leg. Postures include prone sleeping with knees tucked up under the chest, hips extended, or in a 'frog's-legs' position.
- In children able to walk, the commonest conditions that present to paediatric orthopaedic clinics are in-toeing and flat feet, though serious causes of flat feet usually affect only older children. Important points in evaluating an in-toeing deformity and flat feet are shown in Table 2.24. Some deformities in this group have been associated with persistence of sitting postures, e.g. cross-legged or 'reverse tailor' (floor sitting, knees bent and legs splayed out/back) positions.
- Achiness in the feet is the typical symptom in young children with torsional leg deformities of significance. If the biomechanical problem is sufficiently severe, shoes can rapidly deform.
- Regional musculoskeletal lesions in children <3 years of age are rare but most inflammatory arthritides can affect foot joints. Pain from an inflamed joint results in a miserable child and a refusal to walk.
- Periosteal pain (hyperostosis) in the tibiae and other long bones occurs in Caffey's disease. There is usually symmetrical limb enlargement in this rare condition, which usually occurs before the baby is 6 months old.

Table 2.24 Common patterns of foot deformity in babies and infants

Deformity	Commonest causes	Features
In-toeing	Metatarsus varus	Presents age 0–3 months or when starts to walk. Examination: forefoot varus only (heel is in neutral or valgus). Over 80% correct without surgery though predicting which will is difficult: 'wait and see until age 3' is appropriate
	Torsional lower limb deformity—medial tibial torsion and/or excessive femoral anteversion	Often related to regular prone knee–chest (fetal) sleeping position in babies and toddlers, and persistently sitting on the floor with legs forward internally rotated and knees bent out/backwards in children (see Fig. 2.21)
	Cerebral palsy	Most often caused by excessive femoral anteversion
	Spinal dysraphism	Rare
Flat feet (pes planus)	Idiopathic or familial, hereditary connective tissue diseases, hindfoot disease: tarsal coalitions, arthritis, tumour, osteochondritis, infection etc.	Very common—often asymptomatic. Children often develop medial arch with time (passive big toe extension or standing on toes often reveals it). It is associated with conditions of general tissue laxity. If it occurs with pain and/or stiff flat feet look for peroneal muscle spasm and hindfoot pathology as the cause
Talipes equinovarus (club-foot)	Idiopathic, spina bifida, spinal dysraphism, tibial dysplasia, cerebral palsy, arthrogryposis	Incidence 1–2:1000 overall. Presents at birth. Idiopathic (aetiology unknown) is commonest. Often a family history. Examination: calf wasting, hindfoot and forefoot in equinus (plantaris) and varus
Pes cavus	Idiopathic, peroneal muscular atrophy	High arch (medial and lateral sides), toe clawing. Associated with neurological disease rarely e.g. Friedrich's ataxia

Taking a history

Ask about the site and quality of the pain

- Lower leg pain may be due to one of the causes of 'shin splints', a bone lesion, or algodystrophy.
- Localized anterior lower leg pain occurs in lesions of the anterior tibia e.g. stress fractures, periositis, tibial tubercle osteochondritis, but deeper more diffuse anterior pain (often also medial) occurs in 'shin splints' (see below).
- Minimal or non-traumatic tibial fracture associated with fracture or bony deformity elsewhere raises the possibility of osteogenesis imperfecta.
- Localized or diffuse burning pain suggests a neurogenic cause. In children, disc prolapse is rare. Superficial burning pain may be due to peripheral neuropathy or algodystrophy.
- Algodystrophy typically gives burning pain although it can occur with dull, aching pain or paroxysms. Pain often disturbs sleep. In children it is more common in the lower leg and foot than in the upper limb. Diffuse swelling and skin changes may be present. In many cases trauma is a triggering event but anything from simple sprains to arthroscopic knee surgery can trigger it and 25% are idiopathic cases.
- In children, algodystrophy may occur in the limb distal to an arthritic joint.
- Unremitting, sleep-disturbing pain that is worse on weight-bearing suggests bone or bone marrow pathology e.g. bone tumours, osteomyelitis, or periostitis (hypertrophic osteoarthropathy, Gaucher's disease).

Ask about pain onset during sport

There are typical sports injuries of the lower leg that occur relatively often in active children and adolescents. Ask about pain onset during sport or recurrence during or after specific activities:

- Adolescents may refer to 'shin splints'. Possible conditions include: tibial stress fracture, Osgood–Schlatter's disease, tibialis posterior fasciitis, compartment syndrome, popliteal artery stenosis, and malalignment of the hind- and midfoot.
- Tibial fascial inflammation and pain typically occurs as running begins, though patients can run through it, but it often returns severely after exercise and takes days to wear off. It is associated with hyperpronation of the foot (which increases stretch forces on the tendon).
- Compartment syndrome may be acute (due to muscle necrosis) or chronic. The chronic form occurs almost exclusively in endurance sports. Pain is absent at rest but builds as exercise progresses. It diminishes gradually—usually within a few hours. The pattern of pain and findings from perfusion scintigraphy suggest the cause of pain is ischaemic. Increased compartment pressures can be demonstrated by invasive monitoring.

- Pain from major vessel ischaemia occurs typically with walking. Muscle or a fibrous band in the politeal fossa can compress the popliteal artery.
- Stress fractures occur in young athletes. In girls there may be an association with amenorrhea and generalized osteopenia.

Are there regional traumatic lesions?

In the foot, regional traumatic lesions are quite common, particularly in active children and athletes. Chronic arthritides should be considered:

- Apophysitides (osteochondritides) are quite common (see Table 2.25). Most present with localized pain during exercise. There is tenderness and often swelling and pain on resisted movement of the appropriate tendon.
- Proximal midfoot pain may be caused by an accessory navicular, navicular osteochondritis (Köhler's disease), and tarsal coalitions (abnormal joins between bones leading to joint hypomobility, bilateral in 50% of cases). All lesions may be associated with a rigid flat foot (peroneal spastic flat foot) and will be more painful on weight-bearing.

Table 2.25 Localized painful foot disorders specific to school-age children and adolescents. Tumours are rare but osteoid osteoma should be considered

Site of pain	Disorder	Characteristics of disorder
Posterior heel	Calcaneal apophysitis (Sever's disease)	Traction osteochondritis. Both sexes age 8–10 years
Dorsal midfoot	Accessory navicular	Common finding in all children (50%). In 75% it fuses with main navicular. Majority not painful. Rarely it is associated with exercise-related pain
	Navicular osteochondritis (Köhler's disease).	Boys > girls. Presents with pain, limp and weight bearing on the outside of the foot
	Tarsal coalitions	Asymptomatic or with 'peroneal spastic' (rigid) flat foot (8–16 years)
Medial side of foot (may be diffuse)	Hypermobile flat foot	Children 1–5 years. May have generalized tissue laxity
Lateral side of foot	5th metatarsal base osteochondritis (Iselin's disease)	Children 10–12 years. Possibly due to 2° tendon ossification centre and related to tight shoes
Dorsal and plantar distal midfoot	Stress fracture (rare)	Adolescents—2nd/3rd metatarsal
	Metatarsal head osteochondritis (Freiberg's disease)	Commonly 2nd metatarsal head. Affects active adolescent girls most frequently

- Joint synovitis (pain with immobility-related stiffness) is often difficult to detect clinically. Ankle synovitis is the easiest to be confident about. Soft or springy swelling with tenderness over the dorsal skin crease often suggests an effusion. Synovial thickening can be felt in florid cases circumferentially or just around the lower margins of the malleoli. In oligoarticular JIA the ankle joint is sometimes painlessly swollen.
- Juvenile SpA/ERA is rare in children aged <8, and up until that age oligo/polyarticular JIA is a more likely cause of joint synovitis in the foot. Juvenile SpA/ERA may present with synovitis in a single lower limb joint, enthesitis at the Achilles tendon insertion or plantar fasciitis.
- Dactylitis ('sausage toe') raises the possibility of psoriatic arthritis or sarcoid. History usually discriminates the pattern of arthritis that helps in the differential diagnosis.
- The most common other arthritides to involve foot joints are viral and post-streptococcal arthritis and Lyme disease.
- Diffuse foot swelling occasionally occurs with synovitis in oligo/polyarticular JIA. The major differential is algodystrophy. Both pains are worse at night. Sensory symptoms are prominent and skin changes common in established algodystrophy.
- Forefoot pain in adolescents may be due to an interdigital neuroma (Morton's metatarsalgia) or osteochondritis of a metatarsal head (Freiberg's osteochondritis). Neuroma pain is often associated with dysaesthesia and numbness between the toes.
- Big toe pain from hallux rigidus (<50° passive dorsiflexion) is rare but can occur after injury and prevent running.
- Unlike in adults, gout occurs rarely in children and usually only in the context of renal failure, glucose 6-phosphatase deficiency (von Gierke's), malignancy, or X chromosome-linked disorders of uric acid metabolism.

Examination

Observe the lower legs from front and back whilst the patient is standing:

- Lower leg muscle wasting occurs in hereditary sensorimotor neuropathy (bilateral) and typically accompanies spinal dysraphism. Diffuse muscle hypertrophy might suggest muscular dystrophy.
- Extremity swelling occurs in some forms of JIA, vasculitis (e.g. Henoch–Schönlein purpura (HSP)) and sepsis.
- Note the appearance and distribution of any rashes. Skin conditions from venous abnormalities are common. Other skin lesions which may be relevant include purpura (?HSP) and panniculitis over the shins (?erythema nodosum/sarcoid).

Observe the feet from front and back whilst the patient is standing

- Look for swelling and patterns of deformity. Patterns of deformity may require detailed orthopaedic assessment. Check the gait.
- Look for localized oedema—an occasional sign of underlying JIA but also present in nephrotic syndrome and in systemic vasculitides.
- Some torsional leg deformities are clinically significant. The commonest pattern is with the hip internally rotated (usually excessive femoral

anteversion), the tibia compensating in external rotation, and associated hindfoot valgus and forefoot varus.
- Torsional deformities will not spontaneously correct if they've not done so by the age of 7. There is speculation (based on the rationale of joint incongruity), but no proof, that torsional deformities in children are a risk for early OA.
- Flat feet are often asymptomatic and familial, and regress as the child grows (the medial arch becomes evident standing on tiptoe and with passive big toe dorsiflexion). Hindfoot pathology may be a cause.

Examine the sitting patient

With the patient sitting on the edge of the couch, check for tibial torsion:
- Tibial torsion is measured as the angle between an imaginary line through the tibial tubercle in the sagittal plane and the perpendicular of an imaginary line through the malleoli (see Fig. 2.21).

Examine the supine patient

With the patient supine on the couch, examine the lower leg:
- Check for bruising, swelling, and tenderness around the fibular head in patients with foot drop (?peroneal nerve palsy).
- Localized anterior tibial tenderness is often found in patients with stress fractures.
- The purpuric rash of HSP invariably occurs over the back of the calves.

Examine for swellings in the foot
- Bony lumps (exostoses) that may have formed at sites of pressure (e.g. posterior heel—'pump bump').
- Swelling, skin erythema and localized tenderness suggests infection, although synovitis, skin vasculitis and panniculitis (e.g. erythema nodosum) should also be considered.

Examine the hindfoot

In the hindfoot, examine for joint and tendon synovitis, palpate specific structures, and test passive hindfoot joint mobility:
- Synovitis of hindfoot joints is not always easily detected. With ankle joint synovitis thickened tissue may be felt anteriorly in the ankle crease (where there may be a 'springy fullness') or laterally around the malleoli.
- The pain of plantar fasciitis may be elicited by firm palpation of the medial underside of the calcaneum. ERA should be ruled out.
- Posterior tibial and peroneal tendonitis are associated with soft tissue swelling of the medial and lateral hindfoot respectively. Synovial thickening from ankle and talocalcaneal joints may also be felt there and synovitis of structures may coexist in JIA or ERA. Resisting a tendon's movement aiming to elicit specific tendon pain may not be a specific test.
- Painful posterior heel structures are usually easily palpated, though pain may be due to a number of causes including Achilles' enthesitis, mechanical damage to the tendon, retrocalcaneal bursitis, and apophysitis.

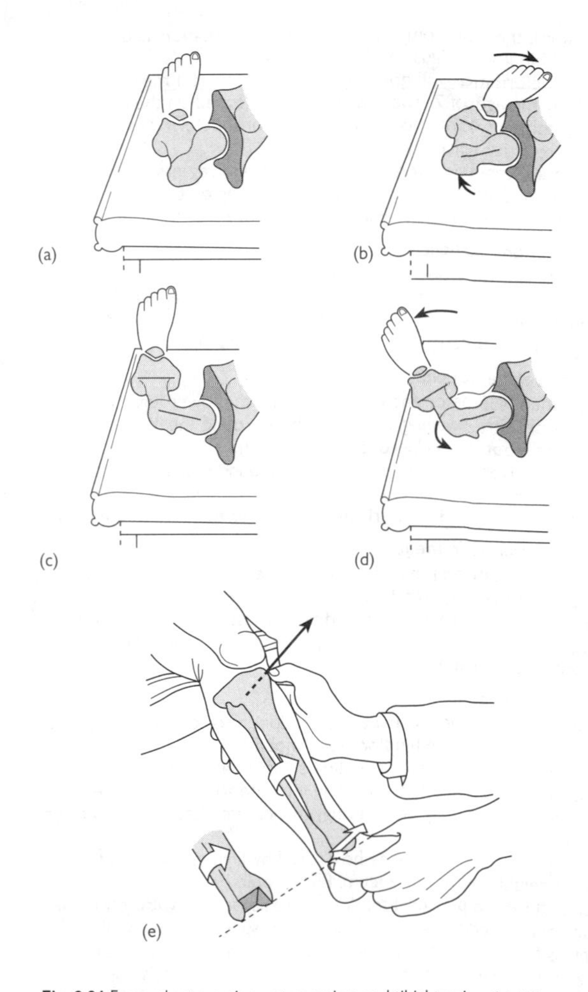

Fig. 2.21 Femoral anteversion, retroversion, and tibial torsion. (a) Where the femoral neck angulates excessively forward relative to an imaginary axis through the femoral condyles, the hip is anteverted. (b) Femoral neck anteversion can lead to a greater than usual range of hip internal rotation and a toe-in gait. (c) and (d) Retroversion, where the femoral neck angulates posteriorly relative to a femoral condyle axis, can cause a toe-out gait. (e) Toeing can also be caused by excessive medial tibial torsion. Normally the ankle mortise faces 15° externally relative to a sagittal plane axis through the tibial tubercle (arrow) but in medial torsion it faces forward or internally.

- The loss of passive hindfoot movements is not specific. Often due to ankle synovitis, stiffness may also occur in other causes of joint pain (e.g. osteochondritis dissecans) and cases of peroneal spastic flat foot. The hindfeet of children are more mobile than those of adults.
- Peroneal 'spastic' (rigid) flat foot syndrome should be distinguished from flexible flat foot (when the medial longitudinal arch reappears when standing on the toes or with passive big toe dorsiflexion). Pain is centred on the dorsomedial side of the foot. The medial longitudinal arch is deficient. Associated peroneal muscle spasm may be painful. The age of presentation depends on the aetiology, the commonest cause being tarsal coalition. It is always important to consider cerebral palsy and spinal dysraphism as well as local lesions: tumours (e.g. osteoid osteoma of calcaneum); navicular osteochondritis (Köhler's); local osteomyelitis or pyogenic arthritis; ankle or talocalcaneal joint synovitis (e.g. JIA). The diagnosis is of underlying cause but AP, lateral, oblique, and axial talocalcaneal radiographs, a three-phase bone scan and hindfoot CT may all be useful in defining associated hindfoot lesions.

Examine the midfoot

In the midfoot determine any sites of tenderness and stiffness:

- Twisting the midfoot may elicit pain from lesions, though non-specifically.
- The major condition to rule out in teenagers is tarsal coalitions. These are fibrous, cartilagenous, or osseous joins between bones resulting in no or little mobility. The commonest involved joints are calcaneonavicular and talocalcaneal. They may be tender. Passive movement with inversion is usually painful and increases spasm in peroneal muscles.
- A tender navicular may also be due to osteochondritis.
- Synovitis associated with some forms of JIA can occur at any joint. Precise location is often difficult to identify clinically.

Examine the forefoot

Check for bony or other swelling, look for digit separation, examine the digits and the sole of the forefoot. Squeezing the whole forefoot at the line of MTPJs is a useful but non-specific screening test for painful forefoot lesions:

- Dactylitis (psoriatic arthritis or sarcoid) swelling is soft, not bony.
- Forefoot splaying and interdigital separation suggests MTPJ synovitis. MTPJs may be tender when palpated (simultaneously with thumb below and finger above).
- Tenderness between two metatarsal heads is typical in Morton's neuroma. The differential (in adolescents) may be osteochondritis of the second or third metatarsal head.
- Extending the big toe passively can reveal an ability to form a medial longitudinal arch in patients with flat feet (Jack's test).
- Discrete bony tenderness without swelling may occur with stress fractures.
- Loss of sensation under the forefoot is rare. Full back and neurological leg examination may be necessary.

Investigations

Imaging of the lower leg

- Radiographs of the lower leg have characteristic patterns of abnormality in osteogenesis imperfecta, rickets, and some periosteal conditions, e.g. from stress fracture or periostitis, etc.
- Bone scintigraphy is a sensitive investigation for radiograph-negative cases of suspected bone disease. It is also a useful initial investigation in adolescents with shin splints as it will rule out stress fractures and can show tibialis fasciitis.
- Treadmill or cycle ergometer exercise scintigraphy using ^{99m}Tc-MIBI can be useful in revealing compartmental perfusion defects in athletes with ischaemic-type pain during exercise (another cause of shin splints).

Imaging of the foot

Local lesions require investigation with radiographs, though in patients with inflammatory or bony lesions further imaging may be necessary:

- Routine AP and lateral hindfoot radiographs will reveal most cases of Sever's disease and osteochondritis dissecans of the ankle. Some cases of talocalcaneal coalition will require extra views and CT for diagnosis.
- In patients with a rigid flat foot additional oblique and axial view radiographs of the hindfoot help to show osteoarticular abnormalities if routine AP and lateral views do not. The gold-standard investigation is CT which is used prior to, and to plan, surgery.
- Forefoot radiographs are a good screening test in those with forefoot pain. Though insensitive for detecting early synovitis, osteochondritides, hallux abnormalities, and the pattern of established arthritis can be identified.
- It is important to check a radiograph for first MTPJ osteochondritis dissecans in those with hallux rigidus.
- Isolated soft tissue swelling may be due to algodystrophy, underlying synovitis, or infection. Radiographs are mandatory. Bone scintigraphy may be non-specific in this setting though the three-phase pattern of abnormality is characteristic in algodystrophy if synovitis can be ruled out.
- MR of the whole foot or swollen area is the quickest way to an advanced differential diagnosis.
- Where swelling, pain, and tenderness coexist infection must be ruled out using imaging. If it cannot and suspicion remains, tissue or fluid sampling should be undertaken. In most cases it is appropriate to do this under general anaesthesia. Algodystrophy should be excluded before any intervention.

Laboratory tests

Any possibility of joint synovitis (most likely to be ankle), enthesitis, tendonitis, or infection requires investigation with laboratory tests:

- ESR and CRP are likely to be raised in cases of autoimmune arthritis and infection and are more likely to be normal or only slightly ↑ in oligoarticular JIA and juvenile ERA compared with polyarticular and systemic JIA or infection.

- Normochromic anaemia (± mild microcytosis) is a non-specific sign of a systemic condition. FBC/CBC may be normal in oligoarticular JIA. Leucoctosis is typical with infection, with steroids and in systemic JIA.
- Moderately ↑ titres of ANA may be present in 40–75% of patients with oligoarticular JIA and is a risk factor for associated uveitis that is not necessarily acute and painful but left unchecked can still threaten sight.
- Check for circulating rheumatoid factor (RF) in cases of synovitis. High titres are a necessary part of, though not specific for, (RF+) polyarticular JIA.

Treatment

Lower leg disorders

- Anterior shin pain should be treated according to cause.
- Treat foot alignment problems with appropriate orthotics.
- Avoid NSAIDs if possible.
- Review diagnosis if conservative treatment fails, e.g. is there an underlying stress fracture or periostitis? (get a bone scan if not already done).

Ankle and foot disorders

- The management of bony anomalies/deformities should be discussed with an orthopedic surgeon and physiotherapist early, to avoid missing an opportunity to prevent growth abnormalities.
- Be aware that soft-tissue steroid injection of a presumed local lesion may impair healing/growth at apophyses and may aggravate the symptoms of (missed) algodystrophy.
- Consider intra-articular steroid injection of specific joints in oligoarticular JIA if joints can be clearly identified by scintigraphy or MR. Injection under sedation (adolescents) or light general anaesthesia (toddlers/children) is appropriate.

Corticosteroid injection therapy

Background

- Local anaesthetic and steroid injection into joints or soft tissues is a very effective treatment for localized pain.
- Injection offers a local maximal anti-inflammatory effect with minimal systemic absorption.
- The indications for local steroid injection include: to reduce inflammation in joints, entheses, tendon sheaths and bursae; to relieve pain from inflammatory ligament lesions; to relieve any inflammation at sites of nerve compression; to attempt to reduce the size of nodules and ganglia; to relieve pain at trigger points; and as part of epidurals.
- The contraindications are:
  - Absolute:
    —septic arthritis/septicaemia
    —febrile patient, cause unknown
    —serious allergy to previous injection
    —sickle cell disease
  - Relative
    —unknown cause of monoarthritis
    —neutropenia, thrombocytopenia
    —anticoagulation or bleeding disorder.
- Hydrocortisone acetate is a short-acting, weak anti-inflammatory, useful for superficial lesions such as tendons and bursae. A dose of 25mg is typical.
- Methylprednisolone acetate (40mg/ml), prednisolone acetate (25mg/ml), and triamcinolone acetonide (10 and 40mg/ml) are long-acting synthetic agents suitable for joint injections.
- Small joints accept only a small volume thus for IPJs, MCPJs, MTPJs, ACJs, and TMJs, 0.5 ml of triamcinolone acetonide (10mg) is appropriate. All other joints should accept at least 1ml. Choice of strength of steroid remains empirical. There may be merit in diluting the steroid in sterile saline, to increase volume for better distribution in larger joints.
- The patient should be warned of potential, though uncommon, side-effects:
  - exacerbation of pain for 24–48 h
  - septic arthritis and reactivation of TB
  - tissue atrophy (less likely with hydrocortisone than others)
  - depigmentation
  - anaphylaxis
  - nerve damage
  - tendon rupture
  - avascular necrosis
  - cartilage damage
  - soft-tissue calcification
  - temporary exacerbation of glycaemia in diabetes.
- As a general rule it is recommended that any one joint should not be injected > four times in 12 months and there are at least 6 weeks between injections.

- Children and some adolescents usually require a light general anaesthetic for most joint injections given the procedure can be quite traumatic. An alternative for older or more robust children or those who have had many injections done before, is to use local anaesthetic gel pads to numb skin adequately before the injection.

Principles of injection techniques

The procedure need not necessarily be done in a sterile environment. Some steps below illustrate the need to maintain relatively aseptic conditions:

- Mark the exact spot of needle insertion.
- Wash hands. Use gloves for procedure (preferably sterile).
- Clean the skin with alcohol.
- Anaesthetize the skin (either with local anaesthetic or refrigerant alcohol spray).
- Insert clean needle with empty syringe and aspirate back.
- Leave needle in place, detach syringe and place syringe containing drug onto end of needle.
- Pull back syringe plunger again before injecting—to ensure not in vein etc.
- Introduction of steroid should be effortless. Resistance implies wrong space.
- On completion remove syringe and needle and throw away 'sharps'.
- Cover the injection site with clean gauze or elastoplast.
- Rest joint for 24h (consider up to 48h for a weight-bearing joint) and re-emphasize possible side-effects and benefits.

The glenohumeral joint

- The anterior route gives reliable access in patients with adhesive capsulitis. It is also better suited for aspiration of joint effusions.
- Palpate the coracoid process anteriorly and the acromion posteriorly. The injection is made just lateral to the coracoid with the needle pointing towards the acromion.
- The posterior route requires the clinician to palpate the spine of the scapula with the thumb to its lateral end where it bends forward as the acromion. With the forefinger then palpate the coracoid anteriorly. The line between finger and thumb then marks the position of the joint line. The needle is advanced from behind, 1 cm below the acromion, and towards the coracoid. There should be no resistance.
- A slight withdrawal of the needle and its advance upward at about 30° also allows this approach to reach the rotator cuff with the same needle!

Subacromial articulation and acromioclavicular joint

- The subacromial bursa is approached from the lateral side. To inject this space the arm is placed in a neutral position, hanging to the side, and the gap between the acromion and the humeral head is palpated. The needle is directed medially and slightly posterior and not too deep.

- The ACJ is located by following the clavicle laterally. The joint is often tender to palpate. The patient lies supine and a small gauge needle with 0.5 ml of steroid is directed into the joint at about 45° anteriorly.

The elbow joint and periarticular elbow structures

- Lateral humeral epicondylitis is injected with the elbow resting on the examination table and flexed at 90°. This superficial injection is directed at 45° to the end of the common extensor tendon origin. A fair amount of pressure is required for this injection. It is often painful.
- Medial humeral epicondylitis is managed similarly. The needle is directed to the flexor tendon origin. However, care should be taken to avoid the groove just behind the medial epicondyle—the site of the ulnar nerve.
- An olecranon bursa can be aspirated and injected superficially with minimal effort. Needle position is confirmed by the aspiration of fluid.
- The elbow joint is most easily reached by a posterior approach. Place the thumb on the lateral epicondyle and the third finger on the olecranon. The groove between the two fingers identifies the joint line. Inject at 90° to the skin, just above and lateral to the olecranon. Alternatively the radial head can be palpated (with forearm pronation/supination) and the needle sited tangentially just under the capsule (anterolateral approach).

Lesions of the wrist

- The radiocarpal joint is best felt with the patient's hand held palm down and the wrist in slight flexion. A triangular gap is felt between the radius and the carpal bones. The needle is pointed proximally and at 60°.
- The carpal tunnel is injected on the palmar surface of the wrist in the first crease. If the palmaris tendon is present the injection should be sited just medial (i.e. closer to the 'little finger') to the midline, by about 1 cm, and towards the palm at 45°. There should be no resistance on injection or nerve pain.
- De Quervain's tenosynovitis should be injected at the point of maximal tenderness, tangentially along the line of the tendon sheath.

The hand

- The small joints of the hand will normally only accept 0.5–1 ml of injected fluid.
- It is important to remember that the joint line of an MCPJ is about 1 cm distal to the crest of the knuckle. The approach to a PIPJ is from the lateral side.
- PIPJs and DIPJs are often difficult to inject. Accuracy of needle placement within a joint space might be improved by using US guidance.
- Efficacy may be greater using US-guided injection though as yet this is unproved.
- US guidance is mandatory when MCPJs/PIPJs are injected with intra-articular erbium-169 colloid (radiation synovectomy).

Hip joint and periarticular hip lesions

- Hip injection is not a routine outpatient procedure and aspiration and injection under US or fluoroscopic guidance is recommended.
- Meralgia paraesthetica occurs as a consequence of lateral cutaneous nerve entrapment (see p.101) as it traverses the fascia 10cm below and medial to the anterior superior iliac spine. If this spot can be clearly demarcated because of localized tenderness, steroid injection has a greater chance of success.
- The ischial tuberosities are located deep in the medial side of the buttocks. The overlying bursae can become inflamed, causing pain on sitting. These tender points can be injected. The differential diagnosis is enthesitis or possibly coccydinia.
- The coccyx can be palpated centrally (with the patient prone or lying on their side). This site is also amenable to local anaesthetic and steroid injections.
- Adductor apophysitis occurring from a sports injury can be injected simply although it can be difficult to access. An inflamed symphysis pubis is best injected under US guidance.
- Trochanteric bursitis or enthesitis at the greater trochanter can be injected with the patient lying on their good side. The injection site can be very deep and to reduce the risk of fat atrophy from a 'blind approach', it is reasonable to try using hydrocortisone first. Injection failure should raise the possibility of poor needle position or a different diagnosis, e.g. gluteus medius muscle tear at its insertion or pain referred from a lumbosacral disorder.

The knee joint and periarticular lesions

- The most common technique for injection of the knee joint is either the lateral or medial retropatellar approach.
- From the lateral side, the joint line is marked between the upper and middle third of the patella. Access to the joint space may be improved by depressing the medial aspect of the patella, tipping it up laterally. The needle is advanced tangentially between the patella and the femoral condyle.
- The entry site for the medial approach is below the midline of the patella, with the needle advanced tangentially towards the suprapatellar pouch.
- In both techniques, aspiration as the needle is inserted will reveal fluid as soon as the capsule is entered, so reducing the risk of forcing the needle too far forward causing cartilage damage.
- Prepatellar bursitis, painful ligaments, and trigger points around the knee may all respond to local steroid and anaesthetic.
- Popliteal cysts can be directly aspirated and injected but owing to the risk of damaging superficial neurovascular structures, should be done under US guidance.

Ankle and foot disorders

- The ankle joint is located most easily with the patient supine on a couch. The joint line can be palpated just lateral to the extensor digitorum tendon as it crosses the ankle crease. The needle is initially advanced downwards over the talus.

- Tendon sheaths and the tarsal tunnel can all be injected; the latter is injected under the flexor retinaculum between the calcaneum and the medial malleolus.
- Painful points under the heel should be injected from the medial side after carefully localizing the position of maximal pain. Never inject through the sole of the foot. Some clinicians will numb the area by local anaesthetic to the posterior tibial nerve, in the tarsal tunnel.
- The MTPJs are injected from the lateral side. Care should be taken as these joints have a greater than normal risk of infection after the procedure.

Principles of rehabilitation

Adulthood

It is beyond the scope of this book to address the many techniques employed in rehabilitation. The reader is encouraged to discuss and observe the management of patients with arthritis with the rehabilitation 'team'.

- In the last decade the development of a multiprofessional approach to rehabilitation has transformed the way most rheumatologists think about disability.
- Two main types of measurement exist for assessing outcome in rehabilitation (beyond the various scoring systems for particular diseases).
- 'Generic' measures take a global view of disability and afford later comparison. Generic measures also help in assessing different programmes, populations, and practices. 'Specific' measures deal with the individual patient and their function in their own environment.
- No one instrument will suffice and there are now many, some well-validated, disability scores:
  - Ritchie index—impairment
  - Health Assessment Qustionnaire—disability
  - SF36
  - General Health Questionnaire—quality of life
  - Nottingham Health Profile
  - Beck depression score—depression
  - Spielberg score—anxiety
  - Sickness Impact Profile (SIP)
  - Multi-dimensional pain inventory—psychological response to pain and disability.
- Important components of rehabilitation for patients with arthritis include:
  - a coordinated team
  - problem-solving approach
  - functionally relevant programme
  - education
  - community orientated
  - cognitive and psychological behavioral therapy
  - addressing social factors e.g. work, housing etc.
  - access to support services
  - commitment to long-term follow-up and reassessment.
- As such the team will consist of doctors, specialist nurses, physiotherapists, occupational therapists, counsellors, psychologists, orthotists, chiropodists, dieticians, rehabilitation engineers, and social workers.

Childhood

There are important additional issues to consider in the management of children:

- A child's rheumatic disease always has an impact on their family. Many normal activities are impossible or time-consuming, and financial hardship is common.
- Siblings may feel neglected and parents are often overburdened with tasks and worries to focus completely on the family. The 'team' aims to share out that burden and assist the whole family.

- The child should be integrated in school ('mainstream' preferably) and social life as much as possible. It is important to achieve the highest level of integration, hopefully ceasing a child's perception of sickness and difference, acquiring a sense of belonging and purpose.
- The therapist will spend as much time preventing deformity in early disease as dealing with chronic disability, the aim being to maintain or restore function.
- For a child with chronic progressive disease a regular, often daily, therapy programme is necessary. The best way to guarantee this is to involve the parents or carer. With education on the role of splints/exercise and the impact of rehabilitation on disease progression, most parents are eager and capable participants in the therapy.
- Joint protection training is important—proper positioning, use of several joints in a task, safe transfer of loads, avoidance of prolonged position, planning of rest breaks, and adapted aids and devices should all be addressed.
- Chronic diseases may elicit different emotions in different children—often frustration with lack of mobility in the young, and peer group issues and psychosexual anxieties in the adolescent. Positive adjustment, focusing on strengths not weakness, is important, as is the constant awareness of such issues in those that make up the support structure. Competence comes in many forms, not simply physical ability, and should be praised at every level, building a child's self-esteem.
- Many children who have learned to cope with their disease develop a more mature personality earlier than others in their age group. As such the adolescent may be earlier and better qualified to bid for an independent life despite physical limitations. It is important to ensure they are not 'held back'.

Adolescence

At some point in a patient's development from childhood to adulthood, the paediatric physician must start to relinquish care to the adult physician. This phase of patient management, the 'transition', should be handled carefully. Some important principles to consider are stated below.

- Transfer should only occur when a young person feels ready to function in an adult clinic.
- From an early stage adolescents should be encouraged to take responsibility for medications.
- The whole concept of independence should be introduced well ahead of an anticipated 'transfer time'. This could be introduced at about the age of 11 years and encouraged by trying to see the adolescent by themselves for part of their consultation by the time they are 13–14 years of age.
- A schedule of events leading to 'transition' and finally to transfer of care should be drawn up.
- Adolescents should be given information on health care rights and taught how to recognize changes in their disease (good or bad) and how to seek help from health professionals.

Chapter 3

Patterns of disease presentation: making a working diagnosis

Oligoarticular pains in adults

Background

The assessment of an inflamed joint

- The clinical features of inflammation and pain at any given synovial joint and the differential diagnosis in the context of other possible regional musculoskeletal diagnoses are discussed in Chapter 2.
- Synovitis is the term given to inflammation of the synovial lining. Inflammation may be a consequence of a range of cellular processes but there are no clinical features that are both frequent and specific enough to allow a reliable diagnosis to be made of its cause in any single joint. Joint effusions (of variable size) invariably accompany synovitis.
- In any given joint, synovitis may not be the only inflamed tissue. Enthesitis of insertions of joint capsules, intra-articular and periarticular ligaments/tendons may be the 1° site of inflammation in some disorders. Subtle differentiating clinical and radiological signs may exist.
- The differential diagnosis of synovitis includes haemarthrosis and other synovial processes, e.g. pigmented villonodular synovitis (PVNS).

Table 3.1 lists the commonest causes of oligoarticular joint pain.

History: general points

- Pain and stiffness are typical though not invariable features of synovitis and enthesitis. Pain and stiffness are often worse during or after a period of immobility. The presence or absence of stiffness does not discriminate between diagnoses. Pain is often severe in acute joint inflammation. In chronic situations, pain may be less severe (e.g. owing to mechanisms which increase physical and psychological tolerance). There are no specific descriptors that discriminate pain from synovitis or enthesitis, although descriptions of 'aching' and 'tightness' are common.
- Swelling, either due to synovial thickening or effusion, often but not always, accompanies synovitis. Enthesitis may be associated with periarticular soft tissue swelling. A patient's report of swelling is not always reliable.
- Reduced mobility in a joint affected by enthesitis/synovitis is almost universal regardless of its cause.

Examination: general points

- Swelling may be observed or detected by palpation. Its absence does not rule out synovitis or enthesitis. Synovial swelling needs to be discriminated from bony swelling, fat, and other connective tissue swellings (e.g. ganglia, nodules, etc.). Without imaging or attempting to aspirate joint fluid, it is often difficult to discriminate synovial thickening from effusion. It is perhaps easiest in the knee.
- Skin erythema (implying periarticular inflammation) and heat do not always accompany joint inflammation but are common with crystal and septic arthritis. Erythema can also occur in reactive arthritis, rheumatic fever and with early Heberden's/Bouchard's nodes in OA.

Table 3.1 The commonest causes of oligoarticular (including monoarticular) joint pain and typical patterns of presentation

Disease	Typical pattern
Gout (Chapter 15)	Age >40 years. Initially acute monoarthritis. Strong association with hyperuricaemia, renal impairment, and diuretics. Possible general symptoms mimicking sepsis. Possible family history. Acute phase often high. Neutrophilia occurs. Joint fluid urate crystals seen by PLM. Joint erosions (radiographically typical) and tophi occur in chronic disease
Spondylarthritis (Chapter 8)	Age <40 years, ♂ > ♀. Mostly oligoarticular lower limb joint enthesitis/synovitis. May occur with sacroiliitis, urethritis or cervicitis, uveitis, gut inflammation, psoriasis (scaly or pustular). Possible family history. ESR/CRP may be normal. More severe course in HLA B27 positive people
CPPD arthritis (Chapter 15)	Mean age 72 years. Oligoarticular, acute monoarticular (25%) and occasionally polyarticular patterns of synovitis
Haemarthrosis	Obvious trauma does not always occur. Swelling usually considerable. Causes include trauma (e.g. cruciate rupture or intra-articular fracture), pigmented villonodular synovitis, bleeding diatheses, and chondrocalcinosis
Osteoarthritis (Chapter 6)	Soft tissue swelling is usually not as obvious as bony swelling (osteophytes). Typical distribution (e.g. first carpometacarpal and knee joints)
Rheumatoid arthritis (Chapter 5)	Unusual presentation in a single joint. Can present with just a few (usually symmetrical) joints
Septic arthritis (excluding *N. gonorrhae*) (Chapter 17)	Commonest cause *Staphylococcus aureus*. Associated with chronic arthritis, joint prostheses, and reduced host immunity. Peak incidence in elderly. Systemic symptoms common and sometimes overt, though may not occur. Synovial fluid is Gram stain positive in 50% of cases and culture positive in 90% of cases
Gonococcal arthritis (Chapter 17)	Age 15–30 in urban populations and with inherited deficiency of complements C5 to C9. One form presents as an acute septic monoarthritis. Organism detected by Gram stain of joint fluid in 25% and by culture in 50% in the second group

- Tenderness of thickened synovium is common but is not always present. Severely tender swelling suggests joint infection, haemarthrosis or an acute inflammatory reaction to crystals. Inflammation of entheses results in 'bony' tenderness at joint margins and sites of tendon or ligament insertion.
- Decreased range of movement is almost always demonstrable in a joint affected by synovitis or enthesitis. The degree to which passive and active joint mobility is reduced depends on a number of often interdependent factors (e.g. pain, size of effusion, periarticular muscle weakness or pain).

- Symptoms elicited by movement of a joint affected by synovitis or enthesitis include pain and stiffness, though neither may be specific. Reaching the end of (reduced) joint range, whether elicited passively or actively, invariably causes pain (though it should be noted that if any normal joint is forced through the end of range, pain can result).

Taking a history

Age, sex, and occupation

The age, sex, and occupation of the patient give non-specific but important clues in many cases:

- Oligoarthritis is uncommon in young adults. SpA, especially reactive arthritis, is likely to be the main cause.
- 75% of patients who develop reactive arthritis are <40 years old.
- Gout typically occurs in those >40 and is the commonest cause of inflammatory arthritis in men (self-reported in 1 in 74 men and 1 in 156 women).
- The mean age of patients with calcium pyrophosphate dihydrate (CPPD) arthritis is about 72 years (range 63–93 years).
- Forestry workers in areas endemic for tick infection with *Borrelia* are at risk of Lyme arthritis.

Which joints are affected?

Some processes are more common in certain joints than others:

- Shoulder synovitis is typical in hydroxyapatite arthritis (Milwaukee shoulder/knee syndrome) and AL amyloidosis.
- Involvement of a shoulder or hip is extremely unusual in gout.
- CPPD arthritis (as pseudogout) occurs rarely in the small finger joints.
- The knee is the commonest site of acute CPPD arthritis and is the site of about 50% of septic and the majority of gonococcal arthritis cases.
- Acute massive swelling of the knee is typical in Lyme arthritis and can occur with septic arthritis. Massive swelling of the knee can also occur in psoriatic arthritis but the history is usually chronic.
- There are many theoretical causes of synovitis in a single first MTPJ but the majority of cases are due to gout (50–70% of first attacks occur in this joint).

Preceding factors

Factors preceding swelling of a single joint or oligoarthritis may be highly relevant. These importantly include infection and trauma:

- Acute non-traumatic monoarticular synovitis is most commonly due to crystal-induced synovitis or associated with SpA.
- A preceding history of trauma typically suggests intra-articular fracture (?haemarthrosis), a meniscus tear (knee), or an intrarticular loose body such as an osteochondral fragment (?locking).
- Twinges of joint pain often precede an acute attack of gout (petit attacks). Acute arthritis occurs in 25% of patients with CPPD arthritis.
- In hydroxyapatite arthritis, synovitis is usually mild-to-moderate, gradual in onset and typically worse at night.
- An acute monoarthritis with fever in familial Mediterranean fever (FMF) is a mimic of septic arthritis. Such joint manifestations are a common (75% of cases) but not invariable feature of the disease.
- ⚠ Septic arthritis should always be considered (and promptly ruled out) as a cause of acute joint swelling.

Crystal arthritides

Crystal arthritides are associated with non-musculoskeletal conditions:

- Hyperuricaemia, causes of which include obesity, renal insufficiency, tumour lysis syndrome, myeloproliferative diseases, and haemolytic anaemia, is associated with gout.
- Hypertension and hypertriglyceridaemia are associated with gout.
- A history of renal stones (urate) may be a clue to hyperuricaemia and associated gout.
- Attacks of gout and CPPD arthritis can be precipitated by any non-specific illness, trauma and surgery. The commonest associated metabolic disorder is hyperparathyroidism (10% of cases).
- Though uncommon, hypomagnesaemia, hypophosphatasia (low ALP activity), haemochromatosis, Wilson's disease, and ochronosis are all associated with CPPD arthritis. The commonest cause of calcium oxalate crystal arthritis (rare) is dialysis-managed end-stage renal disease.

Link with infection

Many types of infection are linked to oligoarticular arthritis. Often a high index of suspicion is needed to make a link:

- Specific infections are directly (joint invasion) and indirectly ('autoimmune reaction') associated with joint synovitis.
- Viruses, bacteria, protozoa, helminthes, and fungi can all directly invade joints. The range of systemic features is wide and pathogens can cause both polyarticular and oligoarticular patterns of joint involvement.
- The infections recognized to trigger reactive arthritis are salmonella, *Yersinia*, *Shigella*, *Campylobacter* and *Chlamydia*. The development of reactive arthritis in those who acquire chlamydial (nongonococcal) urethritis is relatively uncommon (about 1 in 30).
- Acute HIV infection is associated with a subacute oligoarticular arthritis commonly involving knees and ankles.
- Chronic arthritis of any type, diabetes, immunodeficiency, and joint prostheses are risks for septic arthritis.
- Lyme disease should be considered a cause of oligoarthritis in patients with a history (weeks to years ago) of erythema chronicum migrans (macule/papule initially, expanding 0.5–1 cm/day to a mean diameter of 15 cm (range 3–68 cm) fading often without treatment in 3–4 weeks).
- Migratory arthritis is typical in untreated rheumatic fever; however, persistent monoarthritis is a common finding in treated patients.
- A history of circumcorneal eye redness with pain, photophobia, and blurred vision may be due to anterior uveitis most commonly associated with SpA but also sarcoid, Behçet's, and Whipple's disease.

Family and social history

There may be important clues from the family and social history:

- Both gout and SpA may be familial. Between 6–18% of patients with gout have a family history. There may be a family history of SpA or uveitis in patients who have reactive, psoriatic, or enteropathic arthritis or AS.
- Gout in young adults suggests an inherited abnormality (usually ↑ urate production from ↑ 5-phosphoribosyl-1-pyrophosphate synthetase activity, because the other enzyme deficiencies present in childhood).

- Excessive alcohol consumption is associated with gout. Alcohol can also contribute to lactic acidosis that inhibits urate breakdown.
- Consider Lyme disease if patients live, work, or visit endemic areas for infected ticks (within the northeast rural United States, Europe, Russia, China, and Japan). Peak incidence of infection is June/July.
- Brucellar arthritis is generally monoarticular and occurs primarily in areas where domesticated animals are infected and poor methods of animal husbandry, feeding habits, and hygiene standards coexist.

Ask about other (associated) features

Associated extra-articular features include previous eye, gastrointestinal, cardiac, and genitourinary symptoms:

- Low-grade fever, malaise, and anorexia occur commonly in both septic arthritis and gout. Marked fever can occur in gout and only occurs in about a third of patients with septic arthritis.
- Marked fever, hypotension and delirium can occur (rarely) in acute flares of CPPD arthritis.
- Ask about any current or previous features which might suggest SpA: back or buttock pain (enthesitis or sacoiliitis); swelling of a digit (dactylitis); plantar heel pain (plantar fasciitis); red eye with irritation (anterior uveitis); urethritis, balanitis, cervicitis or acute diarrhoea (reactive arthritis); psoriasis; symptoms of inflammatory bowel disease.
- Behçet's disease is a cause of oligoarticular synovitis. Other features include painful oral and genital ulcers and uveitis.
- The involvement of > one joint does not rule out septic arthritis. In up to 20% of cases, multiple joints can become infected.

Examination

General

Review the features (see the beginning of this section) for which you're looking to confirm synovitis in a joint. Always compare sides.

- It is important to establish from the examination whether there is true synovial swelling. A history of swelling is not always reliable and other, non-synovial, pathology can present with single or oligoarticular joint pain. An example might be enthesial inflammation in SpA (though a joint effusion may coexist).

Examine the affected joints

Examine the affected joints for tenderness. Check the range of (passive) movement, for locking and instability:

- Acute processes such as crystal arthritis, infection and post-traumatic effusion often lead to a painful swelling, marked tenderness of swollen soft-tissues, and painfully restricted active and passive movement of the joint. These features are usually less overt with chronic arthritis.
- Instability of an acutely inflamed joint or tests for cartilage damage in the knee may be difficult to demonstrate. Further examination will be necessary after drainage of joint fluid/haemarthrosis.
- Detection of enthesis tenderness around the affected joints or at other sites is a useful clue to the underlying diagnosis of SpA.

Examine other musculoskeletal structures
- Examine the low back and typical sites of bony tenderness—sacroiliitis and enthesitis are common features of SpA.
- Tendonitis is not specific and can often occur in gout, CPPD arthritis, SpA, and gonococcal infection.
- Infection is not always monoarticular.

Look for skin rashes and any inflammation
Oligoarthritis may be part of a systemic inflammatory/infective condition.
- Temperature and tachycardia can occur with some non-infective causes of acute arthritis (e.g. crystal arthritis) though their presence in the context of oligoarticular joint swelling requires exclusion of joint infection.
- Gouty tophi may be seen in the pinnae but also anywhere peripherally. They can be difficult to discriminate clinically from rheumatoid nodules. PLM of material obtained by needle aspiration will be diagnostic for tophi.
- The hallmark of relapsing polychondritis is lobe-sparing, full thickness inflammation of the pinna.
- Mouth ulcers are a typical association of any illness; however, crops or large painful tongue and buccal lesions associated with oligoarticular arthritis suggest Behçet's disease.
- A typical site for the osteitis (tender swelling of bone) of SAPHO syndrome is around the sternum and claviculae.
- Skin erythema over a joint suggests crystal arthritis or infection.
- Associated skin rashes may include erythema nodosum (associated with ankle/knee synovitis in acute sarcoid), the purpuric pustular rashes of Behçet's, gonococcal infection (single pustules), and SAPHO syndrome, erythema marginatum (rheumatic fever), or the rare keratoderma blenhorragica (aggressive-looking rash of the sole of the foot in Reiter's disease).
- Psoriasis may be associated with both synovitis and enthesitis.

Investigations
Doubt about the presence of synovitis can be addressed by obtaining US or MR of the joint(s) in question. At larger joints, both are sensitive investigations for the detection of effusion and synovial thickening. Inflammation at periarticular or capsular entheses can be seen.

Joint aspiration
The most important investigation of a patient with monoarticular synovitis is joint aspiration and prompt examination of fluid. Fluid should be sent in sterile bottles for microscopy and culture:
- Synovial fluid appearances are not specific; however, blood or bloodstaining suggests haemarthrosis from trauma (including the aspiration attempt), a haemorrhagic diathesis, haemangioma, PVNS, synovioma, or occasionally CPPD arthritis.
- Turbidity (↓ clarity) of fluid relates to cellular, crystal, lipid, and fibrinous content and is typical in septic arthritis and acute crystal arthritis mainly owing to the number of polymorphonuclear (PMN) leucocytes.

- Cell counts give some diagnostic guidance but are non-specific (see Table 3.2). There is a high probability of infection or gout if the PMN differential is >90%.
- Joint fluid eosinophilia is not specific.
- Compensated PLM of fluid can discriminate urate (3–20μm in length, needle-shaped and negatively birefringent—blue and then yellow as the red plate compensator is rotated through 90°) and calcium-containing crystals such as calcium pyrophosphate (positively birefringent crystals, typically small and rectangular or rhomboid in shape).
- Lipid and cholesterol crystals are not uncommon in joint fluid samples but their significance is unknown.
- Crystals appearing in synovium less commonly but in typical settings include hydroxyapatite associated with Milwaukee shoulder (and knee) syndrome (alizarin red-S stain positive), calcium oxalate in end-stage renal failure on dialysis (may need scanning electron microscopy), cystine in cystinosis, and xanthine in xanthinosis.
- The presence of crystals in joint fluid does not exclude infection.
- The commonest causes of non-GC septic arthritis in Europe and North America are *Stapylococcus aureus* (40–50%), *Stapylococcus epidermidis* (10–15%), *Streptococcal* species (20%), and Gram-negative bacteria (15%).

Radiographs

Radiographs can confirm an effusion, show characteristic patterns of chondral and bone destruction (e.g. in infection or erosive gout) and can reveal intra-articular calcification associated with CPPD or hydroxapatite arthritis:

- If septic arthritis is suspected radiographs are essential. Patchy osteopenia and loss of bone cortex are cardinal signs.
- 'Punched-out' erosions (within joints or around metaphyses), soft tissue swellings (tophi), and patchy calcification are hallmarks of chronic gout.
- Intra-articular calcification may commonly be either chondrocalcinosis (fine linear or punctate fibrocartilage calcification) or larger loose bodies (often with prolific osteophytes)—both are associated with CPPD arthritis.
- Numerous regularly-shaped calcific masses in a joint may be due to synovial chondromatosis (commonest in middle-aged men, 50% of cases affecting the knee).
- The presence of erosions does not implicate RA. The arthritis may be 2° to an enthesitis associated with SpA.

Further imaging

Further imaging should be discussed with your radiologists:

- MR confirmation of traumatized structures such as meniscus damage in the knee and labral damage in the shoulder should be sought if suspected.
- MR can confirm synovitis, although appearances are usually nonspecific. Characteristic MR appearances of enthesitis and PVNS are recognized.

Table 3.2 Characteristics of joint fluid

Characteristic	Normal	Group I (non-inflammatory)	Group II (inflammatory)	Group III (septic)
Viscosity	Very high	High	Low	Variable
Colour	None	Straw	Straw or opalescent	Variable with organisms
Clarity	Clear	Clear	Translucent or opaque	Opaque
Leucocytes (cells/mm^3)	200	200 2000	2000 50 000	>50 000
PMNs (%)	<25	25	Often >50	>75

Laboratory investigations to consider

- FBC/CBC, acute phase response (ESR, CRP). Neutrophilia is not specific for infection and can occur in crystal arthritis.
- Blood urea, electrolytes, creatinine and urate (e.g. hyperuricaemia and renal impairment associated with gout).
- Blood calcium, phosphate, albumin, ALP (±PTH), thyroid function tests and ferritin to screen for hyperparathyroid or thyroid disease or haemochromatosis associated with CPPD arthritis.
- Autoantibodies: RF may help to characterize an autoimmune process where synovitis is chronic. It is not specific for RA.
- Serum angiotensin converting enzyme (sACE) (i.e. sarcoid), IgM *Borellia burgdorferi* serology (?acute arthropathy or patients with history of migratory arthritris in Lyme disease).
- Antibodies to the streptococcal antigens streptolysin O (ASOT) DNAase B, hyaluronidase, and streptozyme in patients who have had sore throat, migratory arthritis, or features of rheumatic fever.

Synovial biopsy

- If there is a haemarthrosis or suspicion of PVNS, MR of the joint is wise before undertaking a biopsy to characterize the vascularity of a lesion.
- Consider a biopsy in the following situations: undiagnosed monoarthritis, suspicion of: sarcoid arthropathy, infection despite negative synovial fluid microscopy and cultures, gout despite failure to detect crystals in synovial fluid and amyloid (see below).
- Formalin fixation of samples is sufficient in most cases. Samples for PLM are best fixed in alcohol (urate is dissolved out by formalin). Snap freezing in nitrogen is essential if immunohistochemistry is required.
- Arthroscopic biopsy will yield more tissue than needle biopsy, it may add diagnostic information and joint irrigation can be undertaken.
- Congo red staining of synovium, ideally with PLM, should be requested if AA, AL, or β_2-microglobulin amyloid is a possibility. Typical situations are in myeloma (AL) and long-term dialysis patients (β_2-microglobulin). AA amyloid (in long-standing RA, AS, FMF, and Crohn's disease) is a rare though recognized complication of each condition.

Oligoarticular pains in children and adolescents

Background

Disease classification

There has been considerable debate as to the best way of classifying the autoimmune (non-infective, non-reactive) articular disorders in children. The following section aims to help you evaluate conditions that present with one or just a few inflamed joints. In 2001 a working group under the auspices of The International League of Associations for Rheumatology (ILAR) met to establish a consensus regarding classification criteria for paediatric and adolescent arthritides (see below). For a review of these new and old autoimmune arthritis classifications see below and Table 3.4 and under the relevant diagnostic headings in Chapter 7.

Important issues pertinent to children and adolescents

- Compared with the process with adults, it may be quite difficult to establish whether there is synovitis in a child's joint (see Table 3.3).
- An awareness of injurious and mechanical conditions that present at or around specific joints, notably at epiphyseal or apophyseal growth plates, is essential. Prompt investigation in hospital is essential.
- In very young children a history from both the child and parent or main carer is important. It is important to note that monoarticular or oligoarticular synovitis:
  - may present with limb pain
  - may not necessarily present with joint pain and stiffness
  - may result in non-use, altered use, or irritability, any of which may be the main or only complaint.
- Systemic juvenile idiopathic arthritis (JIA) (previously systemic onset juvenile chronic arthritis (JCA)) is proposed to be classified as arthritis preceded by or with daily recurring fever of >2 weeks' duration (documented for >3 days) plus one or more of: an evanescent, non-fixed, erythematous rash; generalized lymphadenopathy; enlarged liver or spleen; serositis.
- Persistent oligoarthritis is proposed to be defined by the involvement of no more than four joints throughout the disease course. Extended oligoarthritis affects a cumulative total of five joints or more after the first 6 months of disease. Excluded from each group will be those with: a family history of psoriasis (first- or second degree relative); a positive RF; HLA B27 (males >8 years old); systemic arthritis.

Table 3.3 The major causes of monoarticular/oligoarticular joint synovitis or swelling in children

Condition	Distinguishing features
Septic arthritis	Systemically unwell child. With TB—pulmonary disease, lower limb, insidious onset, and rapid joint destruction
Trauma	Direct blow/forced hyperextension, haemorrhage into joint
Foreign body synovitis	History of injury
PVNS	Recurrent joint haemarthrosis
Thalassaemia	Episodic and migratory arthritis
Malignancy	Acute monoarticular joint swelling, associated with leukaemia and neuroblastoma
Viral arthritis	Associated with rash or immunization
Lyme disease	Exposure in endemic area, rash, positive serology
Post-streptococcal	Sore throat, migratory arthritis, signs of rheumatic fever
FMF	Ethnic grouping and familial aggregation, acute febrile episode with chest/abdominal pain
Behcet's disease	Rare. Orogenital ulceration and skin rashes
Oligoarticular JIA	Monoarticular in 60% of cases and involves two joints in 31% of cases. Diagnosis of exclusion, associated with asymptomatic uveitis
Enthesitis-related arthritis	Usually age 8 or over, boys > girls, iritis, most have enthesitis, HLA B27. Sacroiliac joint involvement, low back stiffness
Psoriatic arthritis*	Rash, nail pitting, or other changes
Sarcoid	Usually associated with rash and ocular symptoms
Vasculitis	Rash, high ESR/CRP
SLE	UV sensitive skin rash, ANA

* In the new ILAR classifications, psoriatic arthritis is distinguished from enthesitis-related arthritis (see below).

- It is proposed that, enthesitis be adopted to have a key-classifying role in the group of conditions previously classified as spondylarthropathy (SpA), now to be termed enthesitis-related arthritis (ERA).
- The definition of psoriatic arthritis will be broadened under the new ILAR classification (Table 3.4). Enthesitis, iritis and HLA B27 are absent from its proposed classification criteria: arthritis beginning before 16 years of age and either typical psoriasis or at least three of dactylitis, nail pitting, psoriasis-like rash, family history of psoriasis (first- and second-degree relatives). The definitions may be altered further.

Table 3.4 Proposed ILAR classification of arthritis in childhood (juvenile idiopathic arthritis)

ILAR classification of juvenile idiopathic arthritis (JIA)	Previous classification
Systemic arthritis*	Systemic onset JCA
Oligoarthritis* which is either: persistent (always 4 joints or less) extended (after 6 months >4 four joints affected)	Oligoarticular JRA Pauciarticular JCA
Polyarthritis (RF+)* 5 or more joints affected	Polyarticular JRA Polyarticular JCA (RF+)
Polyarthritis (RF–)	Polyarticular JCA (RF–)
Psoriatic arthritis*	Psoriatic arthritis
Enthesitis-related arthritis (ERA)*	SpA

JCA = juvenile chronic arthritis; JRA = juvenile rheumatoid arthritis; RF = rheumatoid factor.
* See text for notes.

Taking a history

Epidemiology

Recall epidemiological features associated with different groups and ages:

- The peak incidence of oligoarticular JIA (or pauciarticular JCA) is between the ages of 1 and 3. It is relatively very rare after 12 years of age.
- Enthesitis-related arthritis (ERA or SpA) is more common in boys (ratio up to 10:1) and typically occurs after the age of 8.
- Familial Mediterranean fever (FMF) can manifest in children as young as 1 year old. There is restriction to ethnic groups in Iraq, Turkey, Libya, Algeria, Morocco, and Tunisia and in Sephardic Jews, and familial aggregation. Acute or chronic oligoarthritis can occur.

Trauma?

Monoarticular synovitis may be associated with trauma:

- Time to onset of joint swelling after trauma (<2 h) and intensity of pain (severe) may help discriminate whether a haemarthrosis is present. Intra-articular fracture should then be suspected.
- An absence of a history of trauma does not rule out the possibility of osteochondritis dissecans (only 10% are associated with trauma).
- Be aware that non-accidental trauma can present with traumatic joint swelling.

Infection/malignancy

Infection and malignancy should be considered as it is a priority that they are ruled out in all cases of atraumatic monoarthritis:

- An insidious onset does not rule out infection. This pattern is well recognized in TB. Joint destruction, however, may not be insidious, therefore don't delay investigation.
- *Haemophilus influenzae* is the commonest cause of septic arthritis in children <5 years and *Staphylococcus aureus* in those >5 years.

- The commonest neoplastic causes of monoarticular joint swelling in children are leukaemia and neuroblastoma.

Rare causes of symptoms

The rarer causes of monoarticular synovitis, joint swelling, or pain, and joint-specific causes of pain in a single joint should be recalled at an early stage:

- Intra-articular haemangiomas, osteoid osteomas, synovial chondromatosis and lipomatosis arborescens can occur in most joints.
- Anterior knee pain in growing adolescents, commonly girls.
- Isolated hip pain conditions such as Perthes'.
- Oligoarticular JIA (Pauci-JCA) of the hip is very rare.
- Osteochondritides/avulsion fractures, e.g. Osgood–Schlatter's.
- Osteonecrosis at typical sites, e.g. tarsal navicular, carpal lunate.

Preceding symptoms

Ask about preceding symptoms of infection and rashes. Consider viral (including vaccinations), streptococcal and enteric infections, and Lyme disease:

- Oligoarthritis (or monoarthritis) may be a reaction to an infection and may be short-lived usually lasting 3–6 weeks, but occasionally up to 8 weeks.
- A streptococcal sore throat can lead on to a migratory arthritis. The differential diagnosis would include rheumatic fever and Lyme disease.
- The most distinctive features of acute rheumatic fever should be sought in patients with oligoarthritis, especially if it has been partially treated with aspirin or NSAIDs which can mask its migratory nature: carditis with prolonged PR interval, chorea, skin nodules, erythema marginatum.
- Salmonella, shigella, yersinia, and campylobacter enteric infections are associated with reactive arthritis.
- *Eschericia coli* and *Clostridium difficile* infections have the potential for triggering reactive arthritis.
- A facial rash occurs in rubella—coalescing erythema that clears as the limbs become affected, and with parvovirus B19 infection (erythema infectiosum—'slapped cheeks').
- Pink or faintly red erythema on the trunk or limbs but not the face is typical of erythema marginatum (rheumatic fever). The outer rash margin is often distinct and continuous. Firm, non-tender skin nodules, which may have regressed, may also suggest rheumatic fever.
- Lyme disease causes erythema chronicum migrans, a spreading erythema from a tick bite.
- Live attenuated rubella vaccines are associated, in up to 15% people, with subsequent joint/muscle symptoms. Arthritis may occur 2 weeks after the injection and clears in a week, but symptoms can remain for a year or so.

Family history

Ask about a history of illness in the family or a family history of enthesitis-related (SpA) features:

- In children suspected of having septic arthritis due to TB, establishing a history of contact with sources may be important.
- Owing to a link with HLA B27, there may be a history of similar musculoskeletal features in family members.

Examination

General principles of paediatric musculoskeletal examination

- Ensure that the child is comfortable in the environment, whilst changing, and with the people present at the time of examination.
- Reassure the child that the examination will not persist if it is painful.
- Observe small children playing at first.
- Try to leave the painful area until last.

Confirmation of synovitis/enthesitis in a joint

Review the features that help to confirm synovitis/enthesitis in a joint:

- It is important to establish from the examination whether there is true synovial swelling. Remember, a history of swelling is not always reliable and other, non-synovial, pathology can present with single or oligoarticular joint pain, e.g. enthesitis.
- Always compare sides. Even subtle differences in joint range may be important and denote synovial thickening.
- Doubt about synovial swelling can be addressed by obtaining US or MR.

Additional musculoskeletal examination

Additional musculoskeletal examination must include a search for muscle atrophy, tenosynovitis, enthesitis tenderness elsewhere, and spinal limitation:

- Adjacent muscle wasting may be a clue to the severity or chronicity of joint inflammation.
- Tenosynovitis is unusual in oligoarticular JIA but can occur in sarcoid, occasionally in ERA/SpA and in the polyarticular conditions.
- Enthesitis should discriminate between oligoarticular JIA and ERA/SpA. Commonly involved sites include Achilles, patellar tendon, and plantar fascia insertions.
- Clinical detection of spinal disease in patients who develop AS or ERA/SpA is not always possible at the time of presentation of the first musculoskeletal manifestations of the disease, i.e. enthesitis, although spinal examination assessing localized pain and impaired mobility should be done.

Look for skin rashes and any inflammation

Oligoarthritis may be part of a systemic inflammatory/infective condition. Look closely for skin rashes:

- Skin erythema overlying a joint suggests infection.
- Associated skin rashes may include erythema nodosum the purpuric pustular rashes of Henoch–Schönlein purpura (HSP) (extensive lower limb) or Behçet's (less florid than HSP), gonococcal infection (single pustules), SAPHO syndrome, erythema marginatum (rheumatic fever) and psoriasis.

Investigations

Although synovitis may be obvious clinically, its presence in any joint needs to be confirmed if there is doubt:

- The soft tissue appearances of joint radiographs are sufficient in confirming effusion and synovial thickening in many instances.
- US and MR can identify effusion and synovial thickening.

Joint aspiration

The most important investigation of a child with monoarticular synovitis is joint aspiration and prompt examination of fluid. Fluid should be sent in sterile bottles for microscopy and culture. This procedure may be psychologically traumatic. Discussion of the case with paediatric colleagues is wise. Consider using sedation (at least) in older children and a light general anaesthetic in younger ones:

- Synovial fluid appearances are not specific. Blood or bloodstaining suggests haemarthrosis from: trauma (including the aspiration), haemorrhagic diathesis, PVNS, synovioma, or haemangioma.
- Turbidity (↓clarity) of fluid relates to cellular, crystal, lipid, and fibrinous content and is typical in septic arthritis and acute crystal arthritis mainly owing to the number of PMNs.
- Crystals in synovial fluid in children are rare.
- The commonest causes of non-gonococcal septic arthritis in Europe and North America are *Staphylococcus aureus* (40–50%), *Staphylococcus epidermidis* (10–15%), streptococcal species (20%), and Gram-negative bacteria (15%). In children <5ys it is *Haemophilus influenzae*. Gonococcal infection should be considered a possibility in teenagers.

Radiographs

Radiographs can confirm an effusion and show characteristic patterns of chondral epiphyseal and bone destruction (e.g. in infection or malignancy):

- In septic arthritis osteopenia and loss of bone cortex are cardinal signs. The main differential diagnosis is malignancy.
- If calcified, loose bodies due to osteochondritis dissecans may be visible.
- The characteristics of tumours/tumour-like lesions can be determined and help decide whether further intervention is necessary.
- Erosions can occur in oligoarticular JIA or in ERA/SpA (enthesial).
- Discriminating erosions from ossifying cartilagenous epiphyses in normal joints (which can appear irregular) is sometimes difficult. Bilateral views are sometimes helpful in this respect.
- Joint space narrowing is difficult to confirm from radiographs because of normal changes in epiphyseal cartilage thickness, projectional errors, and difficulty in weight bearing on painful joints.
- Marked joint destruction is thought to occur primarily in those extending from oligoarticular to polyarticular JIA.

Further imaging

Further imaging should be discussed with your radiologist. US and scintigraphy can confirm synovitis and its pattern of joint involvement. CT and MR are useful in discriminating against the causes of synovitis:

- US is a very sensitive investigation for detection of synovitis and is particularly useful in evaluating the hip.
- US and MR can detect erosions earlier than radiographs.
- Where malignancy and infection are suspected bone scintigraphy is essential for identifying or ruling out additional osseous lesions.

- Because of its high sensitivity, bone scintigraphy can be useful in establishing whether significant bone/joint pathology is present in children with joint symptoms but few clinical findings.
- Bone scintigraphy has a low spatial resolution, thus abnormalities may need further investigation with CT or MR. Therefore, consideration should initially be given to whether the answer to all diagnostic questions can be achieved by proceeding directly to these investigations.
- In a normal joint MR differentiates all the major joint structures including epiphyses. Sedation may be needed in young children.
- MR is an accurate and sensitive tool for identifying joint and epiphyseal damage at an early stage of a disease process. This may be invaluable for example if there is any doubt about the status of oligoarticular JIA or peripheral joint involvement in ERA/SpA as early treatment can then be directed to prevent permanent deformities and disability.

Laboratory tests

Laboratory tests should provide or exclude evidence of infection, give discriminatory diagnostic information, and exclude non-rheumatic diseases:

- FBC/CBC, acute phase response (ESR, CRP). Neutrophilia is compatible with, but not specific for, infection. Monoarticular JIA can be associated with normal indices, however.
- A low platelet or white cell count but ↑ acute phase indices may be suggestive of an underlying malignancy.
- Antibodies to streptolysin O (ASOT) in patients who have had sore throat, migratory arthritis, or features of rheumatic fever. If there is persistent clinical suspicion despite a normal ASOT, antibodies to streptococcal DNAase B, hyaluronidase, and streptozyme may be positive.
- Autoantibodies: a single positive test for RF has little value. Repeatedly positive tests might suggest (RF+) JIA. ANAs are present in 40–75% of children with oligoarticular JIA (JCA). They are not disease-specific but identify a subset within it at particular risk of (often asymptomatic) ureitis.
- Other tests: sACE, Lyme serology (acute arthropathy or patients with history of migratory arthritris).

Synovial biopsy

- If there is a haemarthrosis or suspicion of PVNS, MR of the joint is wise before undertaking biopsy to characterize the vascularity of a lesion.
- Consider a biopsy in the following situations: undiagnosed monoarthritis, suspicion of: sarcoid arthropathy, infection despite negative synovial fluid microscopy and cultures, malignancy.
- Arthroscopic biopsy will yield more tissue than 'blind' needle biopsy. Direct viewing may add diagnostic information and joint irrigation can be undertaken.

Widespread pain in adults

Widespread (musculoskeletal) pain is a common reason for adults to seek medical advice (see Table 3.5). Many conditions are characterized by musculoskeletal symptoms, some of which may be diffuse or multicentric. In addition, the interpretation and reporting of symptoms varies considerably and can be a source of confusion.

Such patients are often referred to rheumatologists in health systems where there is 'gate-keeping' of referral to specialists by primary care physicians. A referral may be made with a working diagnosis in place: 'multiple joint pains, ?rheumatoid arthritis', for example, is a typical comment on such a letter.

In the following section we have aimed to review important aspects of the history, examination, and initial investigations in the diagnostic work-up of patients who present with non-localized, multicentric pains.

Background

Initial impressions

- Think broadly about possible diagnoses from reading any referral letter and whilst meeting the patient.
- Assimilate what you know about the epidemiology of likely conditions. For example, you might reason that the man you are about to see ('age 25 with joint pains') is more likely to have SpA rather than systemic lupus erythematosus (SLE), which occurs mostly in women age 14–50, or PMR which is a condition of the elderly, though joint pains can occur in all.

Age, sex, and racial background

What clues can be drawn from the age, sex, and racial background?

The degree to which these factors influence the likelihood of disease varies according to the background disease occurrence in the (local) population.

- Review what you know about the epidemiology of the major diseases and an appreciation of the limitations of the value of epidemiological data will help you avoid making poor judgements in your diagnostic work-up. Such simple information may prompt the recall of useful data. For example:
  - there is a very low incidence of ankylosing spondylitis (AS) in patients aged >65y with back and joint pains.
  - generalized OA is rare in young men.
  - with an incidence of <1 in a million autoimmune PM is rare compared with PMR which has an incidence of about 1 in 10 000 (age >50 years).
  - SLE is up to five times more common in Black than in White people.
  - osteomalacia occurring in temperate zone 'Western' populations is more likely in economically deprived than in affluent areas, in the institutionalized elderly than in young adults, and in some Asian ethnic groups rather than Caucasians.

Table 3.5 Broad categories of conditions that may present with widespread musculoskeletal pain

Common	Inflammatory polyarthritis (e.g. RA, SpA)
	Generalized (nodal) OA
	Fibromyalgia/chronic pain syndromes
	Non-specific myoarthralgia* associated with infection (e.g. viruses)
Less common	Myoarthralgia* 2° to autoimmune connective tissue disease
	Myalgia 2° muscle inflammation (e.g. polymyositis)
	Myoarthralgia* associated with neoplasia (e.g. lymphoma)
	Skeletal metastases
	Polyostotic Paget's disease
Rare	Metabolic bone diseases (e.g. osteomalacia, renal osteodystrophy)
	Metabolic myopathies (e.g. hypokalaemia)
	Neurological disease (Parkinson's disease)

* In certain situations/conditions patients may complain of both muscle and joint pains. This is easily appreciated if you've ever had influenza! The combination of myalgia and arthralgia is summarized as myoarthralgia.

Previous diagnoses

Presenting features may be put in context early if you have knowledge of musculoskeletal associations of diagnoses that have already been made. For example:

- Synovitis in patients with (radiological) chondrocalcinosis.
- Arthropathy in patients with hyperparathyroidism and hypercalcaemia.
- Enthesitis/synovitis in patients with Crohn's disease or ulcerative colitis.
- Polyarticular synovitis and myalgia in patients with lymphoma.
- Crystal-induced or β_2-microglobulin deposition arthritis and osteodystrophy in chronic renal disease.

Taking a history

Firstly, establish whether pains arise from joints or tendons/entheses, muscles, bone, or are neurological (seeTable 3.5).

- Though the patient or referral letter may report pains as 'joint pains', take care and time to establish where exactly you think the pains arise.
- Listen carefully to the description of the pains that may help discriminate whether the patient has a single condition or a number of causes for pains.

Obtain a detailed history of the pain at different sites

- A good history should give you the anatomical site of pains and should be able to reveal the tissue of origin in the majority of cases. For example, a 70-year-old man referred with 'widespread joint pains mostly in his legs', could have multiple weight-bearing joint OA or, perhaps, lumbosacral nerve root claudication symptoms. In a middle-aged woman with 'hand and neck pain', could the pain be radicular pain associated with cervical spondylosis, or does she have an arthropathy?
- Widespread pain due to bone pathology alone should always be considered and ruled out owing to the possibility of skeletal metastases. Bony pain is often unremitting, day and night. It changes little with changes in posture and movement.
- One pitfall is to assume that all pains arise from a single pathological process. For example, in a retired manual labourer is there PMR or RA causing shoulder, neck, and knee pain or are there different but common causes of the pains such as bilateral subacromial impingement, mechanical neck and upper limb radicular pain, and anterior knee pain owing to patellofemoral OA?

Joint pain at rest, after rest, or with joint use?

How do you establish whether pains arise from joints or tendons/entheses, and are likely to reflect a single process?

- Pain occurring with inflammation is conventionally regarded as being associated with stiffness and worse with immobility, e.g. on waking. It tends to be prominent in conditions such as RA, SpA, PMR, and myositis; however, mild degrees of immobility-associated pain and stiffness occur in some other conditions such as OA and fibromyalgia. Note that stiffness may be a feature of muscle spasm and soft-tissue oedema.
- Mechanical joint damage is also painful. This is typified in OA. Pain may be due to a number of changes in the joint but is usually prominent on weight bearing or use of the joint and rest often eases it.

Ask, and document in detail, which joints are affected

- A symmetrical polyarticular pattern of small joint synovitis is typical of, but not specific for, RA. RA can also present with carpal tunnel syndrome, tenosynovitis, tennis elbow, or an asymmetrical pattern of joint involvement, and can be preceded by a palindromic pattern of joint pain (see below).
- Chronic arthritis from parvovirus B19 infection may also be polyarticular and symmetrical.
- Small hand joint pain occurs in nodal generalized OA. DIPJs and PIPJs and thumb joints are usually affected. Patients often have pain in the spine, hips, and knees owing to changes of OA.
- The combination of sacroiliac (low back and buttock) pelvic, and lower limb joint/enthesis pain, typically in an asymmetrical oligoarticular pattern, is suggestive of SpA. Typical sites include anterior knee, posterior heel and inferior foot (plantar fascia).
- Enthesitis (as the hallmark of SpA) can affect the wrists and small joints of the hand and feet (plantar fascia origin and ?insertion at metatarsal heads) and may be difficult to distinguish from RA on clinical grounds alone.

- Large and medium-sized joints are typically affected in an inflammatory condition 2° to CPPD crystals, but a picture of multiple joint involvement similar to that in RA is possible (including tenosynovitis). CPPD arthritis primarily occurs in old age.
- Widespread arthralgia/arthritis occurs in patients with leukaemias, lymphoma and myeloma and with certain infections.

Ask about the pattern of joint symptoms over time
- A short, striking history of marked, acute polyarticular symptoms often occurs with systemic infection (see Table 3.6). Prominent malaise and fever should raise suspicion of infection.
- There might be a longer history than is first volunteered. Autoimmune rheumatic and connective tissue diseases may evolve over a period of time and often naturally relapse and remit, thus the distribution and severity of joint/tendon/muscle involvement may vary over time.
- Conventionally, persistent inflammatory joint symptoms should be present for at least 6 weeks before RA is diagnosed.
- Migratory arthralgia occurs in 10% of RA patients initially: a single joint becomes inflamed for a few days then improves and a different joint becomes affected for a few days and so on. A similar pattern can occur in post-streptococcal arthritis, occasionally in acute sarcoid, is not unusual before frank oligoarthritis develops in Lyme disease, and occurs in >60% of patients with Whipple's disease.
- The onset of enthesopathy may be insidious or acute—when it can be associated with marked extremity swelling.
- Recurrent pains from various musculoskeletal lesions, which have occurred either from injury or developed insidiously, are typical in patients with underlying hypermobility (benign joint hyper-mobility syndrome or other heritable diseases of connective tissue such as Ehlers–Danlos).

Is there widespread muscle pain?

If you think there is widespread muscle pain, remember to consider that:
- The myalgia may be fibromyalgia or enthesitis.
- Pain locating to muscle group areas may be ischaemic in origin or 2° to neurological disease and not necessarily due to inherent muscle pathology.
- The differential diagnosis of PM and dermatomyositis (DM) is wide though many conditions are rare (see Table 3.7 and Chapter 13).

Ask about the distribution and description of myalgia and weakness
- PMR (rare <50 years), myositis and endocrine/metabolic myopathies typically affect proximal limb and truncal musculature but PMR is also associated with inflammatory polyarthritis and giant cell arteritis (GCA) and therefore may present with headache (for example). In PMR, muscles may characteristically be described as 'stiff' on waking.
- Though rare, truncal muscle pain and stiffness can be a presenting feature of Parkinson's disease.

- Cramp-like pains may be a presenting feature of any myopathy (e.g. hypokalaemic) or even motor neuron disease. However, some patients may interpret radicular (nerve root) pains as 'cramp-like' and therefore explain their presence in a muscular distribution.
- Inflammatory and endocrine/metabolic myopathies are not always painful.
- True weakness may denote either myopathy or a neurological condition. However, patients may report a feeling of weakness if muscles are painful, therefore, rely more on your examination before deciding muscles are weak.
- Occasionally some genetic muscle diseases (e.g. myophosphorylase, acid maltase deficiency), can present atypically late (in adults) with progressive weakness which may be mistaken for PM.

Ask about the pattern of muscle pains over time

- Severe, acute muscle pain occurs in a variety of conditions. The commonest causes are viral, neoplastic, and drugs. Some toxic causes may result in rhabdomyolysis, myoglobinaemia, and renal failure.
- Usually PM/DM is characterized by slowly evolving but progressive muscle pain and weakness (weeks to months).
- In severe, acute presentations consider also the rare eosinophilic fasciitis or eosinophilic-myalgia syndrome (toxic reaction to L-tryptophan).
- Low-grade episodic muscle pains may denote a previously undisclosed hereditary metabolic myopathy.
- Fibromyalgia is chiefly a chronic pain syndrome and symptoms may have been present for a considerable time at presentation.

Are the pains ischaemic?

- Lay persons may have little concept of ischaemia and might describe their symptoms in the context of muscles and in a muscular distribution.
- Ischaemic muscle pain often occurs predictably in association with repeated activity and eases or resolves on rest. Consider this especially if pains are confined to a single limb or both legs.
- The distribution of pains may give clues as to sites of underlying pathology, e.g. upper limbs in subclavian artery stenosis or thoracic outlet syndrome or, typically, thighs and calves in atherosclerotic vascular disease or lumbosacral spine/lumbar nerve root stenosis. Sitting forward may relieve the latter.
- Ischaemic pains in the context of a rash may suggest systemic vasculitis.

Table 3.6 Common infections that can present with acute polyarthritis and a raised acute phase response

Infection	Common extra-articular clinical features	Key laboratory diagnostic tests in acute infection
Rheumatic fever (group A β-haemolytic streptococci)	Acute infection 1–2 weeks earlier, fever, rash, carditis	Positive throat swab culture. High ASCT (in 80%). Anti-DNAaseB IgM
Post-streptococcal (?rheumatic fever)	Acute infection 3–4 weeks earlier, tenosynovitis	As above
Parvovirus B19 (adults[†])	Severe flu-like illness at onset, various rashes	Anti-B19 IgM
Rubella (also post-vaccine)	Fever, coryza, malaise, brief rash	Culture. Anti-rubella IgM
Hepatitis B	Fever, myalgia, malaise, urticaria, abnormal liver function	Bilirubin+, ALT+, AST+, anti-HBsAg, anti-HBcAg
Lyme disease (*Borrelia burgdorferi*)	Tick bites, fever, headache, myalgias, fatigue, nerve palsies	Anti-Bb IgM (ELISA + immunofluorescence)
Toxoplasma gondii	Myositis, parasthesias	Anti-Toxo IgM

Even if serological tests have high sensitivity and specificity, the positive predictive value of the test is low if the clinical likelihood of the infection is low. Therefore, do not use serological tests indiscriminately.

ASOT = anti-streptolysin O titre.

[†]The presentation of parvovirus B19 illness may be quite different in children.

Widespread pain may be due to bone pathology

- Bone pains are unremitting and disturb sleep. They could denote serious pathology—radiographic and laboratory investigations will be important.
- The major diagnoses to consider include disseminated malignancy, multiple myeloma, metabolic bone disease (e.g. renal osteodystrophy, hyperparathyroidism, osteomalacia) and polyostotic Paget's disease.

Past medical history

Specific questions are often required because previous problems may not be regarded as relevant by the patient. For example:

- For those with joint pains a history of the following may be of help: other autoimmune disease (↑ risk of RA, SLE, etc.); Raynaud's phenomenon (association with scleroderma, RA, and SLE); dry eyes (possible Sjögren's syndrome); uveitis or acute 'red eye' (association with SpA); recurrent injuries/joint dislocations (association with hypermobility); genital, urine, or severe gut infection (link with SpA); psoriasis (association with SpA); diabetes (cheirarthropathy).
- For those in whom myalgia/myositis seems likely: preceding viral illness (possible viral myositis); foreign travel (?tropical myositis); other autoimmune disease (associated with PM/DM); previous erythema nodosum, i.e. previous sarcoid (cause of myositis); drugs and substance abuse (see below).
- For all patients: weight loss or anorexia (association with malignancy); temperatures or night sweats (association with infection); sore throat (possible post-streptococcal condition); persistent spinal pain (association with fibromyalgia); rashes (association with Lyme disease, SLE, DM, vasculitis).
- For those with widespread bony pain: history of rickets (association with privational osteomalacia); chronic renal disease (will precede renal osteodystrophy and may predispose to osteoarticular deposition of β_2-microglobulin and crystal arthritides).

Psychosocial and sexual history

- Preceding sexual contact and genital infection is important primarily because of an association of *Chlamydia trachomatis* infection with reactive arthritis and enthesitis/SpA.
- Reactive arthritis has an association with seropositivity of HIV. HIV can itself cause acute PM and is a risk factor for pyomyositis.
- There is an association of anxiety and depression with fibromyalgia.

Ask about travel

- Residence in, or travel to, rural areas populated by deer might be important in indicating a risk of exposure to *Borrelia burgdorferi* and contracting Lyme disease (the spirochaete is carried by ticks which colonize deer, boar, and other animals and bite other mammals).
- *Plasmodium falciparum* (intertropical areas), trypanosoma (mainly South America), trichinella, and cystercercicae infections are associated with myalgia/myositis.

Table 3.7 The major causes of myopathies and conditions associated with diffuse myalgia

Infectious myositis	Viruses (e.g. influenza, hepatitis B or C, coxsackie, HIV, HTLV-I)
	Bacteria (e.g. *Borrelia burgdorferi* (Lyme))
	Other (e.g. malaria toxoplasmosis)
Endocrine and metabolic	Hypo/hyperthyroidism, hypercortisolism, Hyperparathyroidism
	Hypocalcaemic, hypokalaemic
Autoimmune diseases	Polymyositis, dermatomyositis, SLE, scleroderma, Sjögren's, RA, PMR
	Vasculitis (e.g. PAN, Wegener's granulomatosis, rheumatoid)
	Myasthenia gravis
	Eosinophilic fasciitis
Carcinomatous myopathy	
Idiopathic	Fibromyalgia (muscles should not be weak)
	Inclusion body myositis
	Sarcoid myositis
	Eosinophilic-myalgia (L-tryptophan-induced)
Drugs	Lipid-lowering drugs (e.g. lovastatin, clofibrate, gemfibrozil, niacin)
	Anti-immune (e.g. colchicine, CyA, D-Pca*)
	Rhabdomyolysis (e.g. alcohol, opiates)
	Others (e.g. AZT chloroquine*)
Muscular dystrophies	Limb girdle, fascioscapulohumeral
Congenital myopathies†	Mitochondrial myopathy
	Myophosphorylase deficiency Lipid storage diseases

*Drugs most likely to cause painful myopathy.

†Owing to variable severity, some conditions may not present until adulthood.

Note: Guillain–Barré and motor neuron disease may be considered in the differential diagnosis of non-painful muscle weakness.

Family history

Ask about family with arthritis or autoimmune diseases:

- There is an hereditary component to large joint and generalized nodal OA and hyperuricaemia/gout.
- The risk of developing any autoimmune condition is higher in families of patients with autoimmune diseases than generally.

Drug history

- The following drugs have been reported, amongst others, to cause a myopathy (those marked * are more likely to be painful): lithium, chloroquine*, clofibrate, statins, salbutamol, penicillin, colchicine, D-penicillamine*, sulphonamides, hydralazine, cyclosporin, phenytoin, cimetidine* (muscle cramps), zidovudine, carbimazole, and tamoxifen.
- The myositis occurring with D-penicillamine is not dose- or cumulative dose-dependent. It can be life threatening.
- Drug-induced SLE, which is characterized commonly by arthralgia, aching, and malaise, and less commonly by polyarthritis, can occur with a number of drugs including hydralazine, procainamide, isoniazid, and minocycline. Quinidine, labetalol, captopril, phenytoin, methyldopa, and sulphasalazine are among others that probably cause the condition.
- L-tryptophan, which is available as a health food supplement in some countries, has been implicated in causing eosinophilia-myalgia syndrome.
- Mild myoarthralgia may be caused by a number of commonly used drugs, e.g. proton pump inhibitors and quinolone antibiotics.
- Alcohol in excess and some illegal drugs are associated with severe toxic myopathy occasionally resulting in rhabdomyolysis (see Table 3.7).

Ask about chest pain, dyspnoea, palpitations, cough, and haemoptysis

- Cardiac abnormalities are features of autoimmune rheumatic and connective tissue diseases, though infrequent at initial presentation. Cardiac infection is associated with widespread aches and pains (e.g. rheumatic fever/post-streptococcal myoarthralgia, infective endocarditis).
- Chronic effort-related dyspnoea 2° to interstitial lung disease occurs in many patients with autoimmune connective tissue and rheumatic diseases. Up to 40% of RA patients may have CT evidence of lung fibrosis. In the majority of fairly sedentary patients, however, symptoms are not prominent. Dyspnoea may be present at presentation.
- Ventilatory failure and aspiration pneumonia (?postural/nocturnal cough) can occur as a result of a combination of truncal striated, diaphragmatic, and smooth muscle weakness in PM.
- There is an association between bronchiectasis and RA.
- The commonest neoplasm in patients diagnosed with carcinomatous myositis is of the lung.

Ask specifically about dysphagia, abdominal pain, and diarrhoea

- Patients may have overlooked volunteering abdominal and gut symptoms especially if symptoms have resolved. There are many links between bowel disease and polyarthralgia/polyarthritis.
- Ask specifically about previous severe diarrhoeal or dysenteric illnesses, which due to *Campylobacter, Yersinia, Shigella*, or *Salmonella*, may be relevant to diagnosing reactive arthritis/SpA.
- Gut smooth muscle may be affected in PM and give rise to dysphagia and abdominal pain.

Examination

In patients with widespread pain a full medical examination is always necessary.

Skin and nails (see Chapter 4)

In all patients look carefully at the skin and nails:

- Nails may show prominent ridges or pits in psoriatic arthropathy (be suspicious of a previous diagnosis of fungal disease), splinter haemorrhages in infective endocarditis, rheumatoid vasculitis or antiphopholipid syndrome (APS), or periungual erythema.
- Skin rashes in conditions characterized by widespread pain. For example:
  - erythema migrans in Lyme disease
  - erythema marginatum in rheumatic fever
  - UV sensitive rash on face/arms in SLE
  - violacious rash on knuckles/around eyes/base of neck in DM
  - livedo reticularis in SLE and APS
  - purpuric rash in vasculitis (e.g. HSP)
  - erythema nodosum in sarcoidosis.
- Lymphadenopathy may be present with either infection or inflammation and is non-specific. However, if prominent it may denote lymphoma.
- Signs of anaemia are a non-specific finding in many chronic systemic autoimmune diseases.
- Clubbing of the digits may be present in Crohn's disease and ulcerative colitis (associated with SpA) and bronchiectasis (associated with RA).
- Oedema can occur in both upper and lower limb peripheries in a subset of patients presenting with inflammatory polyarthritis/ tenosynovitis. The condition has been termed RS_3PE (remitting seronegative symmetrical synovitis with pitting edema). This condition is striking in that it occurs suddenly, often in patients between 60–80 years old and is very disabling. It may be associated with other conditions e.g. haematologic, malignancy.

Examination of the joints

Important points to note when examining joints (detailed examination techniques that help discriminate synovitis from other pathology at specific joints are included in sections in Chapter 2).

- Each joint should be examined in comparison with its symmetrical partner, firstly by observation, then palpation, then by its active and passive range.
- Useful examination tools include a tape measure for recording swelling (circumferential) and a goniometer (protractor with arms) for measuring the range of joint movement.

Patterns of abnormality

Note the specific cause of joint swelling and site of tenderness, distribution of affected sites, and hypermobility

- In nodal generalized OA, osteophytes (bony swelling—may be tender) can be noted at DIPJs (Heberden's nodes) and PIPJs (Bouchard's nodes). Periosteal new bone at sites of chronic enthesitis may be palpable and tender.

- Nodules may occur in nodal OA, RA, polyarticular gout, multicentric reticulohistiocytosis or hyperlipidaemia (xanthomata).
- Soft tissue swelling with tenderness and painful restriction of the joint on movement suggests inflammatory arthritis. There is often adjacent muscle wasting. This is most easily appreciated in the interossei in small hand joint arthritis or quadriceps in knee arthritis.
- The 'painful joints' may be inflamed tendons or entheses. Tender tendon insertions and periarticular bone tenderness, often without any joint swelling, may denote enthesis inflammation associated with SpA.
- Tendonitis may be part of many autoimmune rheumatic or connective tissue diseases. Look specifically for thickening of the digital flexors and swelling of the dorsal extensor tendon sheath in the hand, and tenderness/swelling of both peroneal and posterior tibial tendons in the foot.
- Gross swelling with painful restriction of small joints is unusual in SLE. Often there is little to find on examination of joints.
- General joint hypermobility may account for, or contribute to, joint and other soft tissue lesions. An examination screen for hypermobility may be helpful (see Table 3.8). Check also for associated features.

Examination of patients with widespread myalgia

- Check for muscle tenderness and weakness. Document the distribution. Is there evidence of neurological or vascular disease?
- As it is common, the characteristic sites of tenderness in fibromyalgia should be confidently recognized (see Fig. 3.1). Despite discomfort, muscles should be strong.
- Examine the strength of both truncal and limb muscle groups (see Fig. 3.2). In the presence of pain it may be difficult to demonstrate subtle degrees of muscle weakness.
- Patterns of muscle weakness are not disease specific; however, there are some characteristic patterns: symmetrical proximal limb and truncal in PM/DM; quadriceps and forearm/finger flexors in inclusion body myositis; limb muscles in mitochondrial myopathy. (Note: using specific apparatus metrologists or physiotherapists can help document isometric muscle strength in certain muscle groups.)
- Muscles in PMR are not intrinsically weak.
- Muscle wasting is not specific. It does not occur in fibromyalgia alone. If wasting is profound and associated with a short history consider neoplasia. Wasting will occur in most long-standing myopathies.
- Check for ↑ limb tone and rigidity—most evident by passive movement at a joint—consistent with extrapyramidal disease. There may be resting tremor in the hand, facial impassivity, and 'stiff' gait. Muscular tone in the limbs may also be ↑ in motor neuron disease (MND); however, if presenting with muscle pains, the patient with MND is more likely to have a lower motor neuron pattern of neuronal loss (progressive muscular atrophy) with muscular weakness/wasting, flaccidity, and fasciculation.
- Diagnostic testing for fatiguability in myasthenia (strictly) requires an examination before and after a placebo-controlled, double-blind injection of an anticholinesterase.

Table 3.8 Features of the benign joint hypermobility syndrome (BJHS).

Examination screen (scored out of 9)	Ability to extend fifth finger >90° at MCPJ (score 1 + 1 for R + L)
	Ability to abduct thumb (with wrist flexion) to touch forearm (score 1 + 1)
	Extension of elbows >10° (1 + 1)
	Extension of knees >10° (1 + 1)
	Ability to place hands flat on floor when standing with knees extended (1)
Associated features	Prolonged arthralgia
	Skin striae, hyperextensibility, and abnormal scarring
	Recurrent joint dislocations
	Varicose veins
	Uterine/rectal prolapse
	Recurrent soft-tissue lesions
	Marfanoid habitus (span > height)
	Eye signs: drooping eyelids, myopia, down-slanting eyes

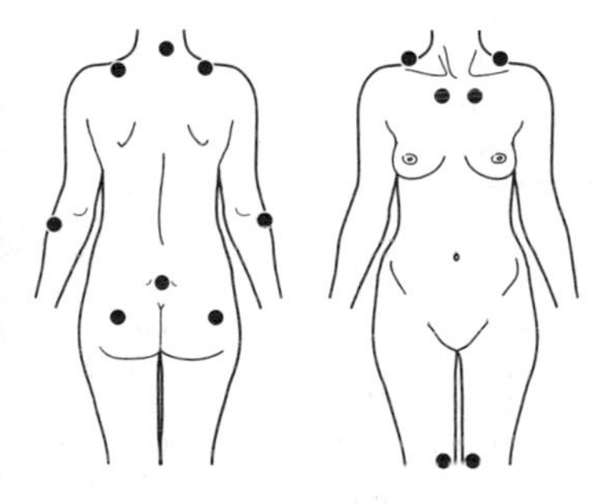

- Tenderness of skin overlaying trapezius
- Low cervical spine
- Midpoint of trapezius
- Supraspinatus
- Pectoralis, maximal lateral to the second costochondral junction
- Lateral epicondyle of the elbow
- Upper gluteal area
- Low lumbar spine
- Medial fat pad of the knee

Fig. 3.1 Typical sites of tenderness in fibromyalgia

- Muscle pains/cramps owing to large-vessel ischaemia are likely to be non-tender at rest and strong. Demonstrate absent pulses and bruits and substantiate findings with US Doppler examination.
- In suspected cases of PM/DM examine carefully for cardiorespiratory abnormalities. Other associated signs in DM include periungual erythema/telangiectasias, erythematous violacious rash and skin calcinosis; include dysphonia and swallowing abnormalities in both PM and DM.
- Because of its associations (see Table 3.7), patients with myositis should be carefully examined for the following signs: dry eyes/mouth (Sjögren's), skin thickening/tenderness or discoloration (scleroderma), skin rashes (SLE), thyroid tenderness/enlargement (endocrine myopathy).

Investigations

General points

- ESR and CRP may be raised in either infection or autoimmune connective tissue or rheumatic diseases. A slightly ↑ ESR is a common finding in healthy elderly people.
- ANA may occur in association with many autoimmune conditions, in other diseases (see Table 3.9) and in some healthy people. It is, therefore, not diagnostic for SLE or any single condition; however, high-titre ANA is often significant and, from a converse perspective, SLE without ANA is rare (immunofluorescence on Hep2 cells).
- RF is not specific for RA. Testing for it will result in little helpful diagnostic information as 1 in 6 people with any infection or an inflammatory condition produce detectable RFs.
- Controversy exists about the diagnosis of fibromyalgia. It is prudent only to make a diagnosis of fibromyalgia in the presence of normal ESR/CRP, FBC (CBC), urea, electrolytes, liver function, and thyroid function tests and if enthesitis can be confidently excluded. Blood calcium, phosphate, serum immunoglobulins and protein electrophoresis may reasonably be added to this list.

Basic tests in patients with polyarthropathy

- Urinalysis (dipstick) may show proteinuria or haematuria. Both glomerular and tubular damage are possible. Glomerulonephritis (in SLE, vasculitis, or endocarditis for example) is usually associated with significant proteinuria (quantified from a 24h urine collection). These patients will need urgent specialist attention.
- ESR and CRP are often raised in autoimmune rheumatic/connective tissue diseases though are non-specific and may be normal in the early stages of these conditions. If very high (e.g. ESR >100) be suspicious of infection or malignancy. ESR >50 is one diagnostic criterion of giant cell arteritis. ESR ↑ slightly in OA but is usually normal. There is often no evidence of an acute phase response in patients with enthesitis (even though pain and bony tenderness may be widespread). FBC (CBC): a mild normochromic normocytic anaemia often accompanies autoimmune connective tissue or rheumatic diseases (e.g. RA, SLE, PMR) infections and malignancy.
- Throat swab, ASOT, anti-DNAaseB antibodies (post-streptococcal condition).

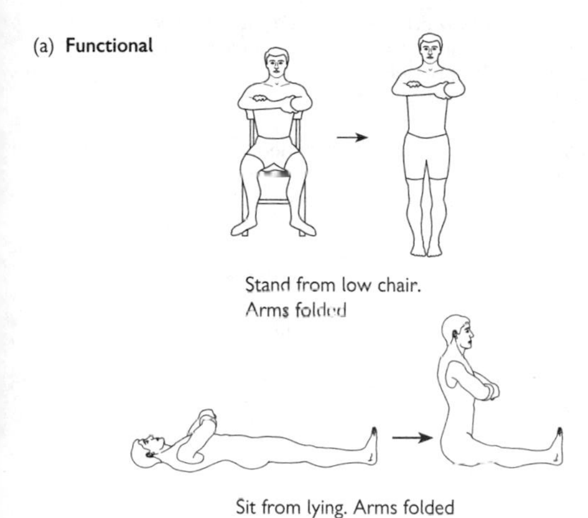

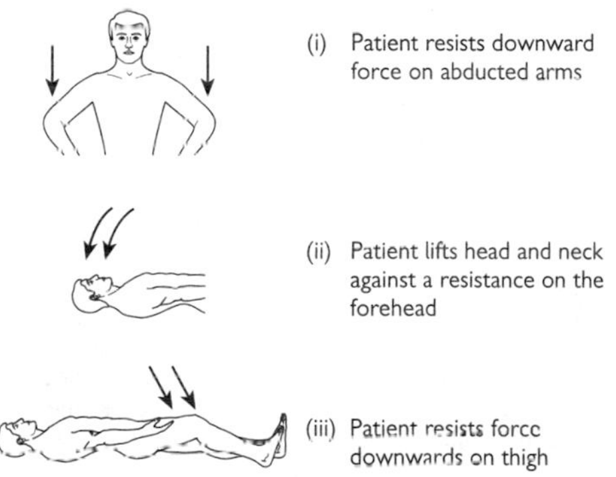

Fig. 3.2 Screening examination for proximal myopathy. (a) Functional movements requiring truncal and proximal lower limb muscle strength. (b) Resisted movement testing of deltoid (i), longitudinal flexors of the neck (ii), and iliospsoas/quadriceps (iii) strength

- Other simple blood tests which should be considered given appropriate clinical evidence for the relevant disease: random blood sugar (diabetes); TFTs/thyroid antibodies (hyper/hypothyroidism); LFTs, prostatic specific antigen (malignancy).
- Joint fluid aspiration and culture is mandatory for patients in whom sepsis is a possibility. Fluid should be examined by PLM in suspected cases of crystal-induced synovitis.
- Testing serum for extractable nuclear antigens (ENAs) may be useful for characterizing the type of autoimmune process. None should be considered alone to be diagnostic or specific for any disease, although diagnostic information is available from certain positive or negative associations.
- Radiographs. In many patients presenting with a short history of widespread joint pains, radiographs may be normal. An early sign of joint inflammation is periarticular osteopenia, though this will not be specific, for example, for RA. Recognized types of erosions and their distribution can be noted by experienced radiologists in specific conditions (e.g. RA, psoriatic arthritis, gout).
- Referral to a sexual health clinic for further detailed investigations if there is a suggestion of recent or recurrent genital infection may help to strengthen the evidence for a diagnosis of reactive arthritis.

Basic laboratory tests in patients with widespread muscle pain/weakness

- Dipstick urinalysis: to screen for haematuria or myoglobinuria.
- FBC (CBC) and measures of acute-phase response.
- An endocrine and metabolic screen: urea/electrolytes, creatinine, thyroxine and TSH, blood calcium, phosphate and 25-hydroxyvitamin D, LFTs.
- Elevated CK occurs in most cases of PM. CK, ALT, AST, LDH, are non-specific markers of muscle damage. Note that specific muscle isoenzymes of CK and LDH exist and the normal range of all enzymes may vary in different populations probably mainly as a function of muscle bulk (e.g. Afro-Caribbean > Caucasian). Muscle enzymes may be elevated after non-inflammatory causes of muscle damage, e.g. exercise/trauma.
- Check for ANA and, if positive, screen for ENAs. Antibodies to certain (cytoplasmic) tRNA synthetases (e.g. Jo-1) are myositis-specific.
- All of the above tests may reasonably be done in cases where you think muscle pains are due to fibromyalgia but want to rule out other pathology.
- Think of checking for urinary myoglobin in cases where acute widespread muscle pain may be associated with excessive alcohol or ingestion of certain drugs (cocaine, amphetamines, ecstacy, heroin), exercise, or trauma. Patients will be at risk of renal failure.
- PM can be the presenting feature of HIV disease thus consider testing HIV serology. In HIV-positive patients, infections causing muscle disease include TB and microsporidia.
- Viral myositis is often clinically indistinguishable from PM. On occasions serology and PCR of muscle tissue/inflammatory cells may reveal diagnostic clues.

Table 3.9 Examples of the prevalence of antinuclear antibodies (ANA) in some diseases using Hep2 cells as substrate

Population group		Prevalence of ANA
Normal population		8%
SLE		95%
Other autoimmune rheumatic diseases •	Systemic sclerosis	90%
	Sjögren's syndrome	80%
	Rheumatoid arthritis	60%
	Polymyositis	40%
	Polarteritis nodosa	18%
Other diseases	Chronic active hepatitis	100%
	Drug-induced lupus	100%
	Myasthenia gravis	50%
	Waldenstrom's macroglobulinaemia	20%
	Diabetes	25%

Electrophysiology and imaging in patients with muscle conditions

- Electromyographic abnormalities occur in two-thirds of patients with muscle inflammation. More information is likely if studied in the acute rather than the chronic phase of the illness. In the acute condition denervation and muscle degeneration give rise to fibrillation potentials in 74% of PM and 33% of DM patients. Other features include: low-amplitude short-duration motor unit and polyphasic potentials.
- Electromyography is poor at discriminating on-going muscle inflammation in myositis from steroid-induced myopathy.
- There are characteristic MR patterns of abnormality in PM/DM. Images can be used to identify potential muscle biopsy sites to avoid false-negative results associated with patchy muscle inflammation.

Muscle biopsy

- With sizeable tissue samples from affected muscle and the judicious application of a range of laboratory techniques, important diagnostic information can be provided. Differential diagnosis needs to be discussed with the pathologist whilst planning the biopsy.
- Myositis may be patchy and biopsy may miss affected muscle. MR is sensitive in identifying areas of muscle inflammation.
- In PM inflammatory infiltrates predominate in the endomysial area around muscle fibres without perifascicular atrophy. In DM inflammation is more prominent in the perimysial area and around small blood vessels and there is typically perifascicular atrophy.
- Routine tests do not reliably distinguish PM from cases of viral myositis. Some of the glycogenoses will become obviously apparent from light microscopy of biopsy material.

Investigations for malignancy

Investigations in adults with widespread bony pain should aim to rule out malignancy, particularly myeloma and 2° malignancies from breast, renal and prostate cancers:

- Investigations may include: breast US/mammography/MR, urine cytology, PSA, renal US, serum and urinary protein electrophoresis.
- Hypercalcaemia may accompany these conditions, thus check blood calcium, phosphate and albumin (also PTH).
- PTH should also be checked in suspected cases of osteomalacia (raised 2° to calcium/vitamin D deficiency) together with 25-hydroxyvitamin D levels (low or low/normal), ALP (high/normal), and 24h urinary calcium (low).
- Radiographs of affected sites are important. Include a CXR.
- Bone scintigraphy can identify sites of neoplasia, Paget's disease, polyostotic osteoporosis or osteomalacia, but although characteristic patterns exist, it is generally not specific for any condition.
- Bone biopsy (maintained undecalcified by placing sample in 70% alcohol) of affected sites will be diagnostic in some, but not all, cases of osteomalacia, osteoporosis, renal osteodystrophy, malignancy, and Paget's disease as good samples are hard to obtain. The best samples are obtained from a transiliac biopsy. Bone marrow can be aspirated for examination at the same time.

Widespread pain in children and adolescents

Background

Disease classification

A working party, under the auspices of The International League of Associations for Rheumatology (ILAR) met in 2001 to establish a consensus about a unifying classification of arthritis in childhood termed juvenile idiopathic arthritis (JIA). A comparison of old and new classification is shown in Table 3.10.

- Systemic JIA (previously systemic onset JCA) is proposed to be classified as arthritis preceded by or with daily recurring fever of >2 days (documented for >3 days) plus one or more of: an evanescent, non-fixed, erythematous rash; generalized lymphadenopathy; enlarged liver or spleen; serositis.
- Persistent oligoarthritis is defined by the involvement of no more than four joints throughout the disease course. Extended oligoarthritis affects a cumulative total of five joints or more after the first 6 months of disease. Excluded from each group will be those with: a family history of psoriasis (first- or second-degree relative); a positive RF; HLA B27 (male >8 years of age); systemic arthritis.
- The definition of psoriatic arthritis will be broadened under the new ILAR classification. The definitions may be altered further.
- It is proposed that enthesitis be adopted to have a key-classifying role in the group of conditions previously classified as SpA.

Assess the distribution of the pain(s)

Are the pains in a joint distribution? What is their pattern?

- Arthralgias may accompany any infection. In this (common) scenario they are short-lived. Persistent (>6 weeks) joint pains raise the possibility of many other diseases (see Table 3.11).
- Post-streptococcal arthralgias are often migratory. Skin overlying joints often appears red in acute rheumatic fever but not in systemic JIA (systemic onset JCA).
- The presentation of polyarticular JIA (RF+ or RF–) is often profound with several weeks' history of worsening joint stiffness and swelling.
- Stiffening is a prominent associated feature of the joint pain in both (RF+) and (RF–) polyarticular JIA.

Table 3.10 Proposed ILAR classification of arthritis in childhood (juvenile idiopathic arthritis)

ILAR classification of JIA	Previous classifications
Systemic arthritis*	Systemic onset JCA
Oligoarthritis* which is either: persistent (always 4 joints or less) extended (after 6 months >4 four joints affected)	Oligoarticular JRA Pauciarticular JCA
Polyarthritis (RF+)* 5 or more joints affected	Polyarticular JRA Polyarticular JCA (RF+)
Polyarthritis (RF–)	Polyarticular JCA (RF–)
Psoriatic arthritis*	Psoriatic arthritis
Enthesitis-related arthritis*	SpA

JCA = juvenile chronic arthritis; JRA = juvenile rheumatoid arthritis; RF = rheumatoid factor.
* See text for notes.

Table 3.11 The differential diagnosis of (RF–) JIA

Infection (multiple sites in immunodeficiency)	*Staphylococcus* septic arthritis
	Haemophilus influenzae septic arthritis
Reactive to an infectious agent	Parvovirus B19, hepatitis, rubella, rubella vaccination
	Post-streptococcal, rheumatic fever
Autoimmune connective tissue disorders	SLE
	MCTD, overlap syndromes
	Poly/dermatomyositis
Systemic vasculitis syndromes	Kawasaki disease (young child, high fever, desquamating extremity rash)
	Polyarteritis nodosa
	Wegener's granulomatosis
	HSP, Behçet's disease, Familial Mediterranean fever
Sarcoid arthritis (polyarthritis, rash, uveitis)	
Haematological disorders	Sickle cell disease
	Constitutional bleeding disorders
	Acute leukaemia (bone and joint pain)
Other causes	Chronic recurrent multifocal osteomyelitis
	Diabetic cheiroarthropathy

Taking a history

Are the pains myalgic or are they in a muscle distribution?

Differential diagnosis is wide (see Table 3.12):

- Acute viral myositis is distinguished from chronic myositis by its localization to calf muscles, severe pain, and its resolution within 4 weeks.
- Chronic muscle weakness suggests an autoimmune connective tissue disease such as PM/DM. Myalgia and muscle cramps occur in hypothyroidism, uraemia, and electrolyte imbalance. Myalgia is common in paediatric SLE but myopathy occurs rarely (10%).
- Episodic cramping or muscle pain related to exercise in early childhood might reflect muscular dystrophy, congenital myopathy, myotonic disorders, or genetic defects in glycogen or glucose metabolism.
- A pain syndrome (e.g. fibromyalgia) is a diagnosis of exclusion. Enthesitis (ERA) should be carefully excluded.

Is there bone pain?

Do the pains represent bone pain—persistent, deep-seated pains which change little with posture or movement?

- Night-time pain is typical of bony involvement in malignancy or osteomyelitis. Acute lymphoblastic leukaemia, lymphoma, and neuroblastoma are the commonest malignant lesions.
- Achy 'bony' pain around joints may be due to enthesitis. Patients with ERA/SpA can present with enthesitis alone.
- Migratory bone pains are typical in multifocal osteomyelitis.

Is the child with arthritis systemically unwell?

- Malignancy should be ruled out and vasculitis and autoimmune connective tissue diseases considered in all children with persistent polyarthritis or widespread pains who have systemic symptoms.
- Fever is non-specific though is essential to making a diagnosis of systemic JIA (see Fig. 3.3). It is spiking with chills and sweats. Anorexia and weight loss are common. Vasculitis and FMF should be considered in appropriate patients.
- There may be several years between the onset of systemic features and the arthritis of systemic JIA.
- Low-grade fever can often be present in patients with (RF–) JIA but is rare in (RF+) JIA.
- Serositis is typical in systemic JIA but also occurs in SLE.
- In children <1 year, fever and arthralgia raise the possibility of chronic infantile neurological cutaneous and articular (CINCA) syndrome and hyperimmunoglobulin D syndrome.

Table 3.12 Classification of childhood disorders characterized by myalgia and muscle weakness

Muscular dystrophies	X-linked, e.g. Duchenne
	Autosomal dominant, e.g. fascioscapulohumeral
	Autosomal recessive: limb girdle
Congenital myopathies	e.g. myopathic arthrogryposis
Myotonic dystrophy	
Metabolic disorders	Glycogen storage disease, e.g. acid maltase/ phosphorylase/phosphofructokinase deficiency
	Familial periodic paralyses
	2° to endocrinopathies, e.g. Addison's disease, Cushing's disease
Inflammatory diseases	Post-infectious, e.g. viruses—influenza B, coxsackie B, echo, polio
	Autoimmune, e.g. juvenile RA, dermatomyositis, SLE
Genetic abnormalities	Osteogenesis imperfecta
	Ehlers–Danlos
	Mucopolysaccharidoses
Trauma	Physical, e.g. rhabdomyolysis
	Toxic, e.g. snakebite
	Drugs, e.g. steroids, hydroxychloroquine, diuretics
Neurogenic atrophies	Spinal muscular and anterior horn cell dysfunction
	Peripheral nerve, e.g. peroneal muscular atrophy
	Neuromuscular, e.g. congenital myasthenia

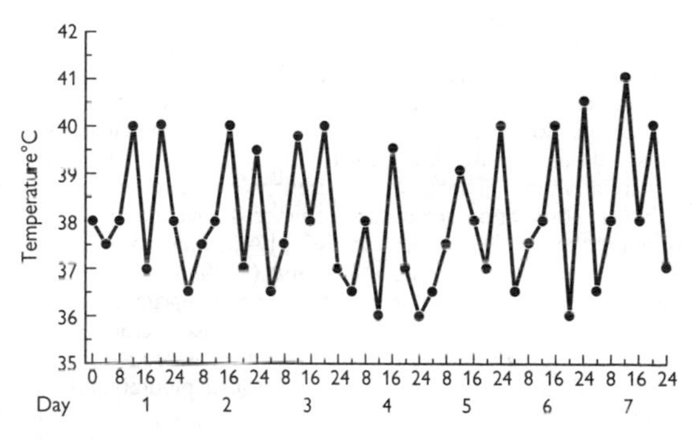

Fig. 3.3 Double daily fever spikes with rapid return to below 37° C in systemic JIA (systemic-onset JCA)

- A catastrophic illness can occur in children with systemic JIA. It is termed macrophage-activation or haemaphagocytic syndrome and is characterized by haemacytopenias, hepatic dysfunction, encephalopathy, and disseminated intravascular coagulation with bleeding.
- A history of recurrent infections and arthritis may suggest immunodeficiency. The commonest is X-linked humoral deficiency.

Is there a rash?

Does the child have a rash or did one precede the onset of pains?

- Rashes raise the possibility of preceding infection: EBV, rubella, and adenovirus are common and are associated with myoarthralgia and fever.
- The rash of systemic JIA is a salmon-pink macular rash. Lesions may either persist or come and go and may exhibit Köebner phenomenon—the exaggeration of the rash at sites of trauma.
- UV skin sensitivity may denote SLE or dermatomyositis.
- Check for a vasculitic rash (e.g. HSP, cutaneous PAN). Systemic vasculitis can be associated with recurrent fevers and joint pains.

Are there ophthalmic symptoms?

Eye symptoms are an important indicator of underlying autoimmunity in the context of persistent joint or muscle pains:

- Uveitis is associated with most forms of JIA (particularly in association with ANA), but also may indicate an ERA/SpA (uveitis = pain/discomfort, blurring of vision, photophobia and a 'red eye').
- Impairment of visual fields suggests a retinal abnormality—a typical manifestation in juvenile DM (due to occlusive vasculopathy).

Examination

Full medical examination

A full medical examination is essential:

- Pharyngeal erythema is non-specific and swabs should be cultured for streptococci. Sterile pharyngitis is a known feature of systemic JIA.
- Lymphadenopathy is common but non-specific.
- For skin examination in detail see pp.204–8. UV sensitivity occurs in DM and SLE; healing psoriasis may mimic Gottron's lesions; calcinosis and pretibial hypopigmentation are signs of DM.
- Cardiovascular examination is important. Pericarditis is common in systemic and other forms of JIA but is infrequently detected clinically. Myocarditis and heart failure also occur (rarely) in systemic JIA. Persistent tachycardia without anaemia/fever raises the possibility of myocarditis. Cardiac conduction defects are common in juvenile DM.
- A variety of cardiac conditions occur in (RF+) JIA including aortic valve insufficiency. The latter also occurs in ERA/SpA (8–30%).
- Respiratory examination may be abnormal if the arthralgia/arthritis is associated with respiratory tract infection; however, fixed crackles may indicate fibrosis (e.g. (RF+) JIA, PM) and a simultaneous reduction in expansion, breath sounds, and vocal fremitus suggests pleural effusion (e.g. (RF+) JIA).

- Bedside eye examination may be unrevealing even in those with ophthalmic symptoms. Retinal vascular changes and field defects might suggest PM/DM. Thrombosis of dilated blood vessels at the margin of the upper lid is characteristic in PM/DM. Eyes may be dry (Shirmer's tear test <5 mm after 5 min) non-specifically in association with autoimmunity.
- As with all chronic conditions of childhood, growth and maturation (skeletal, endocrine/pubertal, and psychological) assessments should be considered at regular intervals.

Musculoskeletal examination—general principles

- Synovitis of a joint is characterized by soft-tissue swelling, effusion, and a reduced range of joint movement.
- Enthesitis around or within joints may coexist with effusion but alone may be represented by tenderness at bony insertions of ligaments/tendons with joint stiffness but without swelling.
- Tendonitis can be difficult to distinguish from synovitis. Its diagnosis requires a precise knowledge of anatomy. The inflamed tendon may be painful on: passive stretch, movement against (an examiner's) directional resistance, and during its normal function.
- If the condition is chronic an assessment of limb growth should be done, e.g. measuring leg length discrepancy.

Musculoskeletal examination—patterns of joint, tendon, and enthesis involvement

A full examination should be undertaken.

- Ligament/tendon insertion tenderness, not necessarily associated with swelling, may denote enthesitis. Enthesitis, which is probably more common, or at least more commonly recognized in lower limbs, raises the possibility of ERA/SpA.
- Within 2 years of onset of symptoms most cases of systemic JIA would be termed oligoarticular because few joints are typically affected initially though often the disease extends to involve more joints. Almost any joint can be involved, including those in the cervical spine. Hip joint involvement is almost always symmetrical.
- There is no consistent pattern of joint or tendon involvement that distinguishes polyarticular (RF+) JIA from the majority of conditions associated with, or characterized by, polyarticular (RF–) JIA.
- Subsets of polyarticular (RF–) arthritis have been suggested on the basis of features such as 'painful' or 'dry' synovitis, stiffness, and other laboratory and genetic indices.
- Muscle tenderness is not specific. If confined to the calves consider viral myositis. Weakness can accompany metabolic and endocrine myopathies and is not specific for PM/DM.
- Muscle weakness at rest may be present in children with severe forms of inherited metabolic muscle diseases. Often weakness only becomes apparent after exercise in these conditions (see Table 3.13).

Laboratory investigations

- Laboratory abnormalities are non-specific in polyarticular (RF–) JIA.
- Not unreasonably because of the appearance of RF in association with infections, ILAR criteria propose that significant titres of RF should be demonstrated on two occasions at least 3 months apart to enable a diagnosis of polyarticular (RF+) JIA to be made.
- A range of laboratory investigations is suggested when considering a diagnosis of systemic JIA (Table 3.14).
- Lymphopenia is a hallmark of DM and SLE and makes a diagnosis of any 1° autoimmune arthritis less likely.
- Neutrophilia and thrombocytosis are invariably present and can be marked in systemic JIA whereas leucopenia and thrombocytopenia are uncommon.
- Urinalysis is important in all children with widespread pains and may detect blood or haemoglobinuria in some muscle diseases (actually is myoglobin). Protein and blood may be a sign of underlying kidney inflammation in connective tissue diseases.
- Conventional acute phase markers can be normal in PM/DM. A sensitive indicator (though non-specific) of active disease is von Willebrand factor.
- A raised CK, ALT/AST, or aldolase is a sensitive but not specific sign of autoimmune myositis.
- ANA is not diagnostic but is associated with all autoimmune connective tissue diseases and some JIA subsets. ANA (speckled) is positive in 60–70% of children with PM/DM.
- Additional initial investigations in those suspected of having myopathic pains include bone biochemistry and TFTs.

Imaging investigations: radiographs

- Employ specialist paediatric radiographers/radiologists if possible.
- Proper X-ray beam coning, high-speed intensifying screens, gonadal shielding, and digital radiography all importantly reduce radiation dose.
- Soft tissue swelling and joint-space widening are important, but non-specific, early signs in all the arthritides in young children.
- The most easily recognized early sign of polyarthritis in an older child will be periarticular osteopenia.
- At joints also look for joint space narrowing, erosions, growth abnormalities, subluxation, and ankylosis. All occur at multiple joints in systemic JIA and polyarticular JIA.
- In children with abnormalities in stature/skeletal morphology look for diffuse (?subtle) changes in bone quality and epiphyses.
- Destruction of bone cortex at sites of pain in patients with myalgia, arthralgia, or polysynovitis may suggest malignancy.

Table 3.13 Characteristics of rare inherited causes of muscle pain and/or weakness

Condition	Musculoskeletal features	Other features
Malignant hyperpyrexia (muscle sensitivity to severe physical or metabolic stress)	Acute rigidity and subsequent rhabdomyolysis	Acute—fever. Hyperkalaemia
McArdle's disease (myophosphorylase deficiency)	Painful (temporary) muscle contractures triggered by exercise	Autosomal recessive. Genotypic and phenotypic heterogeneity
Tauri's disease (phosphofructokinase deficiency)	Similar to McArdle's	Haemolytic anaemia (reticulocytosis)
Von Gierke's disease (glucose 6 phosphatase deficiency)	Skeletal myopathy	Hepatomegaly. Growth retardation. Hypoglycaemia. Lactic acidosis
Pompe's disease (acid maltase deficiency)	Severe skeletal muscle weakness and cardiomyopathy	Death in first year
Cori–Forbes disease (debrancher enzyme deficiency)	Variation from severe childhood myopathic to symptomless adult forms	
Mitochondrial myopathies	Severely limited exercise capacity	Dyspnoea. Lactic acidosis

Imaging investigations: US, skeletal MR, and bone scintigraphy

- The role of US is expanding. It is non-invasive, non-ionizing, can be done at the bedside, and is generally accepted well by children.
- With US, cartilagenous forms of bones can be visualized in comparison to radiographs. This is especially advantageous in the hip where femoral head position and abnormal movement can be seen in young children.
- US is very useful in identifying effusion, notably in the hip and discriminating effusion from synovial thickening.
- Bone scintigraphy provides critical information in musculoskeletal pain when radiographs are unrevealing. Though of less use when joints are involved, bone scintigraphy should be considered when pain originates in bone or infection is a possibility.
- CT is a reliable way of documenting sacroiliac disease in children suspected of having ERA (SpA).
- MR has become the imaging of choice, especially where the diagnosis of JIA is not straightforward. It is more sensitive than radiographs in detecting soft-tissue and most bone lesions, particularly those of the bone marrow.
- MR is more sensitive for detecting changes in joints associated with chronic arthritis compared with radiographs. MR should provide diagnostic information if there is doubt about the presence of arthritis in a joint after clinical examination and radiographs.
- The discrimination of synovitis and enthesitis by MR may have implications for the diagnosis of ERA (SpA) compared with JIA.

Investigations of muscle pains

- EMG patterns of abnormality occur in muscular dystrophy, myasthenia gravis, and autoimmune myositis but each is not specific.
- Evidence of an inflammatory myopathy on EMG is not specific to juvenile DM and may be due to a myositic component of another autoimmune connective tissue disease.
- MR can confirm myositis and reveal potential sites of biopsy in what can be a patchy process.

Table 3.14 Useful tests in investigating suspected systemic JIA

In all patients:	FBC (CBC), ESR, CRP
	Renal and liver biochemistry, serum albumin
	Serum immunoglobulins
	Clotting screen
	Blood cultures
	ECG, CXR, abdominal/pelvic US
	ANA
	Bone marrow aspiration and biopsy
	Ocular slit-lamp examination
	Joint aspirate (single joint)
	Radiographs of selected affected joints
In selected patients:	Muscle enzymes (CK, ALT/AST, and aldolase)
	RF
	Isotope bone/gallium scan
	Upper GI series/small bowel follow-through
	Tissue biopsies
	Viral serology—parvovirus, adenovirus, others
	Echocardiogram
	ASO/antihyaluronidase antibodies
	Urinary homovanillic/vanillylmandelic acid
	Serum IgD

Chapter 4

The spectrum of presentation of rheumatic disease

Skin disorders and rheumatic disease

The importance of examining the skin

- The skin is the most accessible organ to examine.
- Pattern recognition of skin symptoms and lesions is valuable in aiding diagnosis (e.g. acute or chronic sarcoid) and prognosis of rheumatic diseases (e.g. nodules and vasculitis in RA).
- Musculoskeletal abnormalities may be mirrored by skin abnormalities, e.g. joint hypermobility and skin laxity with bruising, scarring, and striae.
- Some anti-rheumatic drugs produce highly specific and potentially serious reactions that require prompt diagnosis and management.

Regional abnormalities

The scalp

Scalp symptoms and lesions may be subtle:

- Scalp tenderness and the description of scalp 'lumps' is recognized in giant cell arteritis.
- C2 root/occipital neuropathy (e.g. in RA) or shingles may be associated with dysaesthesiae over the scalp and occipital neuralgia.
- Alopecia may be localized (areata) or diffuse (e.g. in SLE or iron deficiency). Scarring alopecia is typical of discoid lupus.
- Scalp psoriasis may be patchy and discrete.

Face and ears

Face and ears are in sun-exposed areas. Consider UV skin sensitivity:

- A variety of patterns of SLE-associated, UV-sensitive rashes may occur. The rash is often diffuse. Shaded areas (e.g. nasolabial folds) may not be affected.
- As in SLE, rosacea can present with telangiectatic papules. Distinction is sometimes difficult without biopsy.
- Periorbital oedema occurs in dermatomyositis (?heliotrope rash), angioedema (may be a presenting feature of SLE), and in nephrotic syndrome.
- Heliotrope rash refers to violaceous oedema/erythema of eyelids in dermatomyositis.
- The cutaneous infiltration of chronic sarcoid (lupus pernio) across the nose and cheeks may be overt (papular) but also may be quite subtle.
- Saddle nose deformity/nasal cartilage destruction has a number of causes: Wegener's granulomatosis (WG), relapsing polychondritis, or hereditary connective tissue disease (e.g. Stickler's syndrome.
- Oral aphthous ulcers are common. Oral ulceration may follow disease activity (e.g. in SLE). Ulcers in sexually acquired reactive arthritis are typically painless.
- Large punched-out and numerous tongue and buccal ulcers which scar are a hallmark of Behçet's disease. They may remain for several weeks.

- The strawberry erythema of tongue and lips should not be missed in children. It may denote self-limiting streptococcal infections but may also herald the desquamating palmar (and sole) rash of Kawasaki disease.
- Lacy white streaks on the buccal mucosa suggest lichen planus.
- The pinna is a common site for gouty tophi and discoid lupus. Relapsing polychondritis typically causes softening and distortion of cartilage.
- Lipid skin deposits around the eye occur in hyperlipidaemia and multicentric reticulohistiocytosis.

Hands and nails

Hands and nails should be examined closely:

- A photosensitive eruption spares the finger webs and palms.
- Erythema on the back of fingers may help distinguish dermatomyositis from SLE.
- In patients with Raynaud's phenomenon (RP), finger ulceration, finger pulp atrophy, induration and tethering of skin indicates scleroderma.
- Onycholysis, pitting, salmon patches, and subungual hyperkeratosis are typical of psoriasis.
- Subungual splinter haemorrhages may be associated with trauma, infective endocarditis, systemic vasculitis, or thromboangiitis obliterans.
- Nailfold vasculopathy is non-specific and changes may range from erythema to infarcts. Consider systemic vasculitis, dermatomyositis, and infective endocarditis.
- Nailfold capillaries can be examined with an ophthalmoscope at 40 dioptres applying a drop of oil to the cuticle. Enlarged (dilated) capillary loops and capillary 'dropout' suggests an underlying autoimmune connective tissue disease, particularly SScl.

Types of eruption

Macular rashes

Macular rashes are flat, impalpable areas of altered skin colour. Papules are lumps <1 cm in diameter:

- Maculopapular rashes are typical of viral infections.
- A short-lived pinkish, maculopapular eruption occurs on the trunk and limbs in Still's disease. It is often marked in the late afternoon coinciding with fever. If scratched the rash may blanch ('Koebner phenomenon').
- Erythema that enlarges to form large figurative patches in hours suggests rheumatic fever.
- A spreading area of erythema from an original bite may be erythema chronicum migrans—Lyme disease.
- Maculopapular eruptions can occur from NSAIDs, gold, D-penicillamine, sulphasalazine, azathioprine hypersensitivity, and leflunomide.

Pustules and blisters

Blisters may be vesicles (<0.5 cm diameter) or bullae (>0.5 cm diameter):

- The commonest pustular rash is due to folliculitis.
- Pustules confined to the hands and feet suggest Reiter's, though local forms of psoriasis may be indistinguishable. Psoriasis can also occur as 'raindrop' erythematous lesions (guttate lesions).
- Generalized pustular rashes can occur in vasculitis, intestinal bypass syndromes, Behçet's disease, and gonococcal bacteraemia.
- Bullous eruptions are most likely to be due to SLE and drug reactions in rheumatological practice.

Plaques

Plaques are slightly raised, circumscribed areas of skin, often disc shaped:

- Plaques are the hallmark of psoriasis. Skin may be scaly and flake off easily. Lesions are often red.
- Psoriatic plaque lesions can occur anywhere on the skin but typical sites are over the extensor surfaces of joints, in the natal cleft, and the umbilicus.
- Scaling may be a feature of discoid lupus. The flakiness tends to be at the periphery of the lesion.

Bleeding into the skin

Bleeding into the skin, which does not blanch is termed purpura. It may sometimes be palpable. Telangiectasias are dilated small vascular lesions that blanch on pressure:

- Impalpable purpura may be due to thrombocytopenia, platelet function disorders, trauma (± capillary/skin fragility, e.g. chronic steroid use), haemophilia and hereditary connective tissue diseases (e.g. Ehlers-Danlos).
- Palpable purpura suggests vasculitis including drug-induced.
- Widespread telangiectasias occur in limited cutaneous SScl (lcSScl), hereditary haemorrhagic telangiectasia, and DM.

Ulcers and ulcerating rashes

Ulcers are defined as a loss or defect of dermis and epidermis produced by sloughing of necrotic tissue:

- Cutaneous ulceration may have more than one cause in autoimmune diseases. Vasculitis, venous hypertension in an immobile patient, and ulceration over nodules or pressure points where trauma may be relevant, may all be important.
- An indurated, expanding plum-coloured plaque or acneiform pustule, which then ulcerates, suggests pyoderma gangrenosum. The crater has irregular, bluish margins.
- Neurotropic ulceration occurs rarely in RA. More commonly it occurs in mononeuritis multiplex in association with vasculitis, autoimmune connective tissue disease, or syringomyelia.
- Severe widespread ulceration developing rapidly in a child may suggest dermatomyositis.
- Vasculitic ulcers in the context of livedo reticularis and antibodies to phospholipids (e.g. cardiolipin) may denote antiphospholipid syndrome (APS).

Textural abnormalities

Abnormalities of the texture of the skin may be difficult to discern. Atrophy and thinning, laxity, thickening, and induration may all be associated with disease:

- Generalized skin atrophy and thinning is an age-related process though may be marked at any age in association with chronic steroid use (or at injection sites) and with some heritable diseases of connective tissue.
- Skin laxity can best be demonstrated over elbow and knee extensor surfaces. Generalized laxity of connective tissue may result in varicose veins and internal organ prolapse.
- True acral and digital puffiness in a patient with Raynaud's is suggestive of SScl. Skin thickening has a variety of causes (see below). SScl and scleroderma-like skin may be localized or in a limited or a generalized distribution—distinction is important (see Table 4.1).

Diagnostic issues in patients with skin thickening

- Raynaud's phenomenon (RP) invariably precedes the onset of SScl but is not typical in morphoea or linear scleroderma.
- In patients with RP, abnormal nailfold capillaries on capillaroscopy are a predictive sign of progression to SScl.
- The specificities of autoantibodies are often predictive of SScl subtype. In patients with RP, ANA has predictive value for identifying patients who may progress to SScl; anti-centromere antibody can predict progression to lcSScl; anti-topoisomerase I (Scl-70) and anti-RNA polymerase antibodies are linked to progression to diffuse cutaneous SScl (dcSScl).
- Patients with dcSScl have a preponderance of visceral organ involvement in the first 5 years of disease and screening investigations are usually useful (barium studies of gut, echocardiography, lung function tests, biochemical assessment of liver and renal function).
- Eosinophilic fasciitis is a recognized paraneoplastic syndrome. Haematological malignancies are over-represented.
- Linear scleroderma in children can produce lifelong deformities owing to failure of limbs to develop correct length and bulk.
- Scleroderma-like syndromes may occur secondarily to exposure to some industrial chemicals: vinyl chloride, chlorinated organic solvents, and silicon and epoxy resins.

Table 4.1 Pattern recognition in patients with skin thickening

Classification	Skin features
Morphoea may be localized (guttate) or generalized	Early small skin areas affected (itchy). Progression to hidebound skin, typically on trunk (areola spared) and legs. Lesions become waxy and hypo/hyperpigmented. Guttate (small <10 mm papules) usually on neck and anterior chest
Linear scleroderma	Linear band-like pattern often in dermatomal distribution. Atrophy of muscles is common. Fixed joint deformities and growth abnormalities can occur
'Coup de sabre'	Linear scleroderma on the face/scalp can be depressed; ivory in appearance. Hemiatrophy can occur
Systemic sclerosis (early)	Early morning 'puffiness' in hands and feet, facial 'tightness'. Non-pitting oedema of intact dermal and epidermal appendages. High degree of suspicion needed
Systemic sclerosis (classic)	Firm, taut, hidebound skin proximal to MCP joints. Skin may be coarse, pigmented, and dry. Epidermal thinning, loss of hair, and sweating can occur. Telangiectasias and skin calcinosis become obvious. Skin creases disappear. Such change proximal to elbows or knees in the limbs or below the clavicles (in those with face and neck involvement) classifies disease as diffuse as opposed to limited systemic sclerosis
Systemic sclerosis (late)	2–15 years after onset of classical phase, skin softens but pigmentation changes remain. Skin becomes atrophic and can ulcerate
Eosinophilic fasciitis	Phases: early—pitting oedema; progressive—*peau d'orange*; late—induration ('woody feel') with venous guttering when limb elevated. Arms and legs most commonly affected but fingers mainly spared. Synovitis and low-grade myositis may occur. Eosinophilia is usually striking but not always present
Lipodermatosclerosis	Fibrotic induration of lower legs associated with venous stasis ('champagne-bottle legs')
Diabetes	Waxy thickening of extremities. Insidious progression. Joints of the hands become stiff, the tendons can thicken. Skin changes proximal to wrist and on the face very unlikely but stiffening of elbow and shoulder joints not uncommon
Dependent lymphoedema	Feet/ankles/lower legs. Often pitting. Chronic presence may give hyperkeratosis. Main causes: R- or L-sided heart failure, renal failure, nephrotic syndrome, and low-protein states

Skin vasculitis in adults

Skin vasculitis in adults

Background

There is a variety of ways in which systemic vasculitis may present, including pyrexia of unknown origin, organ infarction, gastrointestinal bleeding, and high acute phase response in a generally unwell patient. However, a vasculitic skin rash is a relatively common presenting feature of systemic vasculitis and therefore its recognition is important.

When to consider a diagnosis of vasculitis

- Systemic vasculitis is rare. Overall the annual incidence is about 40 per million (UK rural population).
- Vasculitis can follow viral or bacterial illness, can be triggered by drugs, and is associated with malignancy. Such vasculitis is often found to be leucocytoclastic on biopsy. The list of causes is long (see Table 4.2); however, in about 50% of cases no cause may be found.
- Vasculitis may be part of another autoimmune disease as in SLE or RA or a disease may be defined by it, e.g. WG, Churg–Strauss, microscopic polyangiitis.
- The commonest systemic vasculitis is WG (12.5 per million average annual incidence) and skin involvement occurs in up to 50% of patients, but the cumulative incidence of other skin vasculitides implies that WG will not be the commonest cause of most skin vasculitis seen.

Important considerations

The following important points of clinical assessment should be followed in patients with possible vasculitic rashes. Vasculitis may be confined to the skin or may be systemic:

- Take a history to include possible triggering causes such as starting a new drug or having had a recent infection. Is there a risk the patient may have hepatitis B/C or HIV?
- Other autoimmune rheumatic or connective tissue, bowel, or hepatic disease may be relevant.
- Ultimately, malignancy will have to be ruled out as a cause.
- The wheals of urticarial vasculitis last 24–72h and tend to have a burning or painful quality. Patients are at risk of glomerulonephritis and chronic lung disease (recurrent cough and haemoptysis). Lymphadenopathy, uveitis, benign intracranial hypertension, low complement and IgM macroglobulin are associated findings.
- Arthritis occurs in many different conditions and is not specific.
- Oral ulceration is common with vasculitis. Severe orogenital lesions are a hallmark of Behçet's syndrome. Eye lesions, thrombophlebitis and arthritis are frequent. The condition is common in Mediterranean populations.
- Dry eyes and mouth are features common to many conditions. If present with vasculitis consider Sjögren's syndrome, which is associated with RP (21%) and cheek (parotid) swelling (24%).

Table 4.2 Precipitants and associations of hypersensitivity (allergic) small vessel vasculitis

Drugs	Sulphonamides and penicillins, for example—there are many
Infections	Hepatitis B, hepatitis C, HIV
	β haemolytic streptococcus
Foreign protein	e.g. serum sickness
Autoimmune disease	Rheumatoid arthritis
	Sjögren's syndrome (anti-Ro positive)
	Systemic lupus erythematosus
Inflammatory diseases	Sarcoid
	Crohn's disease, ulcerative colitis
	Chronic active hepatitis
Malignancy	Myelo- and lymphoproliferative disorders
	Solid tumours
Cryoglobulinaemia	

- Systemic symptoms are common in the 'systemic vasculitides' (WG, Churg–Strauss, polyarteritis nodosa, and microscopic polyangiitis). The diagnosis relies heavily on the results of investigations in all cases.
- In WG there is often a long history of recurrent symptomology, which may include nasal stuffiness, epistaxis, sinus symptoms, middle ear, or inflammatory eye symptoms.
- Churg–Strauss vasculitis occurs in asthmatics. Often patients have had childhood asthma that has resolved to recur severely. There may be allergic rhinitis.

Systemic vasculitis

⚠ Systemic vasculitis is a life-threatening condition.

Two essential initial tasks are firstly to recognize a rash as vasculitic and secondly to determine whether there is multisystem or internal organ involvement:

- The commonest type of vasculitic skin rash is palpable purpura. Lesions may also be impalpable purpura, urticarial, or livedoid.
- Localized vasculitis such as granuloma faciale or erythema elevatum diutinum rarely present to rheumatologists.
- Aggressive panniculitis and neutrophilic dermatoses can sometime present diagnostic difficulties.
- Panniculitis (e.g. erythema nodosum) is usually regional and is due to subepidermal vasculopathy. There may be atrophy and scarring. A migratory panniculitis is recognized.

- Panniculitis is associated with infections: streptococcus, TB, psittacosis, *Yersinia*, *Salmonella*, leprosy, histoplasmosis, blastomycosis, cat scratch fever, and coccidiomycosis; also with oral contraceptives, pregnancy, IBD, pancreatitis, and sarcoid.
- Sweet's syndrome is a combination of painful erythematous plaques, fever, arthralgia, and leucocytosis. The lesions appear in crops, may be initiated by a variety of traumatic injuries (pathergy) and heal without scars. The condition has reported to be para-neoplastic and associated with pregnancy.

Investigations

Skin biopsy

- Try to discuss the case with the pathologist first.
- Take an elliptical biopsy (10 x 5 mm) unless it is undesirable cosmetically. Punch biopsy is simple to do and is often sufficient.
- Include subcutaneous fat in the biopsy, especially if panniculitis is suspected. It allows easier wound closure too.
- Use a needle to lift the skin sample—this avoids forceps-induced damage.
- Fixing in formalin is appropriate for routine histological staining and diagnosis in most cases.
- Immunofluorescence (IF) is important in suspected SLE and in blistering disorders. The lupus band test is positive in clinically uninvolved skin in 70% of cases (sun-exposed sites best).
- Samples for IF should be snap frozen in liquid N_2 or dry ice or transported immediately to the laboratory, ideally in PBS.

Key examination and investigation steps to determine whether there is internal organ or nerve involvement

- Dipstick urinalysis to check for protein or blood, and urine microscopy to look for cellular casts is important. Blood urea, creatinine and electrolytes should be checked. If there is protein, quantify it with a 24hr collection and obtain nephrological advice.
- Pulmonary evaluation and CXR. Cough, dyspnoea, and haemoptysis may suggest WG or pulmonary vasculitis. If lung nodules or infiltrates are seen on the radiograph obtain lung function tests, a high-resolution CT and advice from a chest physician.
- Abdominal pain, diarrhoea and abdominal tenderness may be common findings and due to a number of causes: in some forms of allergic vasculitis, endothelial lesions can lead to gut bleeding (e.g. HSP); gut infarction (in PAN) and mesenteric panniculitis can lead to an acute abdomen; allergic vasculitis may be triggered by hepatitis B and is associated with chronic active hepatitis and inflammatory bowel disease.
- Parasthesiae and numbness may reflect mononeuritis multiplex due to vasculitis. Symptoms may seem trivial. Obtain nerve conduction tests.
- Laboratory investigations should be thorough (see Table 4.3).
- Further investigations which warrant consideration: CT of upper respiratory tract to show the distribution of disease in WG; angiography in suspected cases of PAN; kidney biopsy in cases where renal inflammation is suggested by investigations. Endoscopy and inflammation scintigraphy in suspected cases of bowel vasculitis.

Table 4.3 Laboratory investigations in patients with suspected vasculitis

Haematology	**FBC (CBC), ESR**
Biochemistry	Urea, electrolytes, creatinine
	Liver function enzymes, serum ACE
	CRP
	Serum and urine protein electrophoresis
Microbiology	Blood cultures
	Hepatitis B and C serology. Consider HIV
	Streptococcal antibodies
Immunology	Immunoglobulins, cryoglobulins, complement
	ANA (ENAs), rheumatoid factor
	ANCA

Skin vasculitis in children and adolescents

Epidemiology

- Classification of childhood vasculitis is difficult. A system that has clinical utility is shown in Table 4.4.
- Statistically the commonest type of vasculitis is likely to be HSP then hypersensitivity angiitis (both leucocytoclastic vasculitides). On a worldwide basis, giant cell arteritis is the third commonest.
- Kawasaki disease (KD) affects primarily the under 5s.
- Though commonest in Japan (150/100 000 under 5s), KD occurs worldwide (3–10/100 000 under 5s in Europe and N America).

Clues from the history

- All vasculitides may be associated with features such as fatigue, fever, gastrointestinal symptoms, lymphadenopathy, and myoarthralgia.
- Drugs or infection are often identifyed as a precipitant of a small vessel leucocytoclastic vasculitis, although links to an infective trigger have also been made in cutaneous polyarteritis (URTI), KD (numerous but lately staphylococcus), giant cell arteritis (TB).
- WG is rare. As in adults, it may be characterized by a limited localized form involving the respiratory tract. Subglottic stenosis, nasal septum disease, and respiratory infections may all have occurred.
- Testicular pain is a rare though fairly specific feature for PAN.
- Abdominal pain is not specific. Gut bleeding can occur in HSP and DM especially.
- Vasculitis associated with FMF is not unknown.

Examination

Characteristic examination features of the rash

- Erythematous rash with swelling progressing to desquamation of palms and soles of the feet is typical of KD.
- Lower limb and buttock palpable purpura is typical of, but not specific for, HSP and hypersensitivity angiitis.
- Skin nodules are not specific but are common in cutaneous polyarteritis and frequently occur in hypersensitivity vasculitis. A nodular, painful rash on the medial sides of the feet is frequent in cutaneous polyarteritis.
- Extensive necrotic and ulcerative rash with notable muscle pains suggests DM. Periungual erythema and both eyelid and nail bed telangiectasias are typical.
- Livedo reticularis is a feature of cutaneous polyarteritis (often with painful skin nodules) but also SLE and antiphospholipid syndrome.

Other typical or specific examination features

- Bilateral conjunctival injection, lip/oral/buccal inflammation, and acute non-purulent cervical lymphadenopathy are typical features of KD.
- The incidence of cardiovascular manifestations is 35% in KD. Murmurs, gallop rhythm, and coronary artery aneurysms (30%) can occur.

Table 4.4 A classification of childhood vasculitis

Polyarteritis	Macroscopic
	Microscopic
Kawasaki disease (mucocutaneous lymph node syndrome)	
Granulomatous vasculitis	Wegener's granulomatosis
	Churg–Strauss vasculitis
Leucocytoclastic vasculitis	Henoch–Schönlein purpura
	Hypersensitivity angiitis
Cutaneous polyarteritis	
Vasculitis and autoimmune connective tissue disease	SLE
	JIA
	Mixed connective tissue disease
	Dermatomyositis
	Scleroderma
Large vessel vasculitis	Giant cell arteritis
	Takayasu's disease
Miscellaneous vasculitides	

- Pulselessness may suggest major vessel vasculitis. The most likely is giant cell arteritis.
- Severe oral aphthous ulceration raises the possibility of Behçet's syndrome. It is rare but does occur in children.

Investigations

- Leucocytosis, thrombocytosis, anaemia, and an acute phase response are typical in all forms of vasculitis and are not specific.
- ECG, echocardiography, and usually coronary angiography are essential in suspected KD.
- Glomerulonephritis is not specific and should be ruled out in all cases (urinalysis, urine microscopy, 24-h urinary protein estimation, and in some cases ^{51}Cr EDTA GFR).
- ANCA is not specific but c-ANCA with antibodies to proteinase 3 in appropriate patients suggests that WG should be suspected.
- Biopsy of the skin rash is a key investigation in all patients though in mild typical cases without gut or renal involvement it may not be necessary in HSP.
- Impaired renal function with nephrotic range proteinuria is an indication for renal biopsy in patients with suspected HSP.
- Renal biopsy may be necessary in polyarteritis and WG. The distinction of microscopic polyarteritis from macroscopic disease relies on the extensive glomerular involvement in the former (focal segmental). Aggressive crescentic glomerulonephritis is a feature of WG.
- The most valuable investigation in patients with suspected macroscopic polyarteritis is hepatic and renal angiography.

Endocrine conditions

Well-characterized musculoskeletal conditions occur in many endocrine disorders. Some are specific, others occur with greater frequency than in the general population. Musculoskeletal manifestations occur either as a result of metabolic disturbances or are influenced by a common link through their autoimmune pathophysiology.

Diabetes

- Dupuytren's contracture, trigger finger, carpal tunnel syndrome (about 15% of diabetics), diffuse idiopathic skeletal hyperostosis (DISH), and adhesive capsulitis are more frequent than in the normal population.
- Some form of tissue or joint hypomobility/stiffness is common (see Table 4.5) and can appear similar to scleroderma. However, histo-pathological differences are recognized. Thus to avoid misdiagnosis, do a skin biopsy.

Table 4.5 Patterns of joint and tissue hypomobility or stiffness in diabetes by reported series. Tissue changes are thought to occur from excessive hydration (a consequence of an excessive local production of sugar alcohols)

Patient series	Major abnormalities	Associations
Diabetics overall	In about 30–40% mainly in long-standing disease: slow decrease in hand mobility; waxy skin thickening ('scleroderma-like')	Occasional lung fibrosis. Microvascular diabetic complications
Adults	55–76% prevalence of joint hypomobility in type 1/type 2 diabetes respectively	Not associated with diabetic complications
Mature onset diabetes (mean 61 years)	Stiffening of connective tissue (assessed in hands)	Diabetic nephropathy
Children with type 1 diabetes	31% had limited joint mobility	None with glycaemic control, retinopathy, or proteinuria
Juvenile and young adult onset (age 1–24 years) diabetes	34% had skin thickening. Changes rarely proximal to MCPJs and never proximal to wrists. Joint contractures in >50%, often third or fourth fingers	No flexor tendon rubs (as seen in scleroderma)

- Hand weakness may be due to diabetic neuropathy and may be mistaken for carpal tunnel syndrome. Neurophysiology tests help discriminate.
- Calcification of soft tissues around the shoulder is common (about 20% of diabetics) but is associated with variable symptoms and disability.
- Amyotrophy is rare. It presents acutely with pain, weakness, and wasting of the proximal lower limb muscles. It may be unilateral. Differential diagnosis includes myositis and polymyalgia rheumatica (PMR). It is associated with uncontrolled hyperglycaemia. Aetiology is unknown but it is probably a neuromyopathy.
- Though rare (1:500 diabetics), neuropathic arthritis can occur in advanced disease. Most patients are aged 40–60 years and have poor glycaemic control. Tarsal and metatarsal joints are most frequently affected (60%). The usual presentation is of swelling of the foot with no or little pain. Trauma may have occurred. Early radiographic changes can resemble OA.
- Asymptomatic osteolysis can occur at the distal metatarsals and proximal phalanges with relative joint sparing. The aetiology is unknown.
- Osteomyelitis is not uncommon and needs to be discriminated from cellulitis and neuropathic arthritis. A three-phase bone scan should be helpful. Osteomyelitis is usually disclosed by prominent blood flow in the dynamic (first) phase and increased uptake of tracer by soft tissue and bone in later stages. Cellulitis is associated with minimal uptake of tracer in bone in the delayed (third) phase. Neuropathic joints display minimal first-phase abnormality but prominent tracer uptake in the third phase.
- Muscle infarction can present as a painful muscle mass and is a result of arterial narrowing. Often mistaken for thrombophlebitis, myositis or vasculitis this is a late complication of diabetes. Biopsy may be needed.
- Insulin resistance is associated with features of autoimmune connective tissue disease such as arthralgia, alopecia, glandular enlargement, ↓WCC, ↑Igs and antinuclear antibodies.

Hypothyroid disease

- Over 25% of patients may have an arthropathy. The arthropathy can be mistaken for RA.
- The commonest arthritis usually involves large joints, especially knees. It is characterized by pain, stiffness, effusions, and synovial thickening. It is not clear whether this inflammatory arthropathy can be ascribed entirely to synovitis caused by calcium pyrophosphate dihydrate deposition (CPPD arthritis—'pseudogout').
- Also a small joint arthropathy occurs. Symptoms are more obvious than signs. A third have flexor tenosynovitis and acroparasthesiae are common.
- Carpal tunnel syndrome is frequent (7%). Up to 10% of patients with carpal tunnel syndrome may have hypothyroidism.

- Chondrocalcinosis (radiographically defined) is only marginally increased compared with controls (17% vs 10%). About 1/10 patients with pseudogout are hypothyroid.
- Hyperuricaemia is common but gout attacks are rare. However, screening for hypothyroidism in patients with gout is recommended. Treated hypothyroidism then requires review of the need for uric acid-lowering therapy.
- Musculoskeletal symptoms are otherwise common with patterns of pain similar to PMR (normal or slightly ↑ESR) or fibromyalgia. Improvement occurs after the thyroid is treated.
- Consequences of hypothyroidism in children included retarded bone age, short stature, and epiphyseal dysgenesis with premature epiphyseal plate closure and chance of slipped femoral epiphyses.
- Myopathy is relatively common. About 1 in 20 cases of acquired myopathy are due to hypothyroidism. Presentation can mimic polymyositis with elevation of muscle enzymes though muscle biopsy typically shows no inflammatory cell infiltrate. Improvement with thyroxine replacement is sometimes complicated by muscle cramps but takes only a few weeks.
- The combination of weakness, muscular stiffness, and an increase in muscle mass in an adult with myxoedema is termed Hoffman's syndrome. Muscle mass increase is sometimes striking and can take many months to resolve on treatment. The same condition occurs in children (Kocher–Debre–Semelaigne syndrome).
- Lymphocytic thyroiditis (Hashimoto's) is an autoimmune condition characterized by hypothyroidism and autoantibodies to thyroglobulin and thyroid microsomes. These antibodies are found in 40% of patients with primary Sjögren's disease but only about 10% are or have been overtly hypothyroid.

Hyperparathyroidism

Unless stated, points refer to both primary and secondary disease:

- Musculoskeletal symptoms are the initial manifestation in up to 16% of patients with primary hyperparathyroidism.
- Hyperparathyroidism, chondrocalcinosis, and pseudogout frequently coexist. Pseudogout (CPPD) can be triggered by parathyroidectomy.
- A polyarthropathy can occur which can mimic RA. It differs in that synovial proliferation is absent. Radiographically, erosions have a predilection for the ulna side of distal upper limb joints (radial in RA), joint space is preserved, pericapsular calcification is often present, and reactive bone formation ultimately occurs.
- A polyarthropathy can occur with renal osteodystrophy in about 20% of patients with chronic renal failure on dialysis. It does not appear to be related to CPPD.
- Hyperparathyroidism is associated with a specific shoulder arthropathy characterized by intra/periarticular erosions of the humeral head. Calcification may be absent and damage subclinical.

- Subjective muscle weakness is common, objective weakness less so. Fatiguability is a common complaint. Muscle enzymes are normal. Biopsy shows type II fibre atrophy and features of an inflammatory myopathy are absent.
- The hallmark of radiographic changes is bone resorption: subperiosteal (typically on the radial side of second and third phalanges), intracortical, subchondral, trabecular, subligamentous, and localized (Brown's tumours). Bone sclerosis, periostitis, and chondrocalcinosis also occur.
- Fragility fracture is common and often precedes a diagnosis of primary hyperparathyroidism. Although significant and fast accretion of bone occurs after surgery, long-term relatively low bone mass often remains.

Thyrotoxicosis

- Hyperthyroidism can cause a proximal myopathy (70%), shoulder periarthritis (7%), acropachy (thickening of extremities), and osteoporosis.
- Acropachy is rare (<2% of patients with thyrotoxicosis) and most often occurs in treated patients who are hypo/euthyroid. It consists of clubbing, painful soft tissue swelling of hands and feet, and periosteal new bone on the radial aspect of the second and third metacarpals.
- Graves' disease is frequently associated with fatiguability and muscular weakness. It is associated with autoimmune rheumatic and connective tissue diseases.

Acromegalic arthropathy

- Over-stimulation of bone and connective tissue cells from excessive growth hormone can result in a multiplicity of features: bursal and cartilage hyperplasia, synovial and bony proliferation, an OA-like picture, backache, and hypermobility.
- Joint complaints usually manifest about 10 years after the onset of clinical acromegaly. Knees are frequently affected.
- Joint symptoms are not typical of an inflammatory arthritis—morning stiffness is not prominent and joint swelling is present in <50% of patients.
- Carpal tunnel syndrome affects >50% of patients and is frequently bilateral.
- Back and neck pain and radicular symptoms from nerve root compression or spinal stenosis are not uncommon and are related to axial bony proliferation.
- A painless proximal myopathy occurs infrequently.
- Radiographs characteristically show widened joint spaces (e.g. >2.5 mm in adult MCPJs) and a thickened heel pad (>23 mm in men and >21.5 mm in women).
- Diagnosis relies on demonstration of a failure of growth hormone to be suppressed by a glucose tolerance test but a lateral skull radiograph is a good screening test as 90% have enlargement of the pituitary fossa.

Gut and hepatobiliary conditions

Musculoskeletal features frequently occur in patients with gut or hepatobiliary disease (see Table 4.6)

- Data on the frequency of rheumatological features are largely based on studies of hospital patients with clinically overt gut or biliary disease. This may lead to an underestimate of the frequency of association.
- The most frequent associations are: sacroiliitis, arthritis and enthesitis in patients with inflammatory bowel disease; inflammatory arthritis in coeliac disease and viral hepatitis; and degenerative arthritis in haemochromatosis and Wilson's disease, for example.
- The frequency of enthesitis in patients with inflammatory bowel disease may be underestimated. Be aware of the easiest sites where inflammation (tenderness) may be detected: medial/lateral humeral epicondyles, Achilles tendon insertion, calcaneal plantar fascia origin and insertion, patellar tendon origin and its insertion at the tibial tubercle.
- Radiological studies in patients with inflammatory bowel disease suggest that sacroiliitis is under-recognized by clinicians.

Severity of rheumatological manifestations

- Optimal surveillance strategies for the musculoskeletal manifestations of gut or biliary disease are not known in many instances.
- Life-threatening vasculitis is associated with hepatitis B or C.
- In most patients who develop joint inflammation or enthesitis after bacterial dysentery, the condition is self-limiting. Chronicity and severity may be linked to HLA B27 prevalence. Progressive spondylitis is rare.

Characteristic gut and hepatobiliary conditions in patients with rheumatological diseases (see Table 4.7)

- The commonest problem in RA patients is dyspepsia associated with gastroduodenal erosions or ulcers due to NSAIDs. Peptic lesions may be clinically silent and may present with dropping haemoglobin levels or an acute bleed.

Table 4.6 Rheumatological features in patients with gut or hepatic disease

Gastrointestinal disorder	Rheumatic manifestation	Association
Enteric infection	Reactive arthritis: self-limiting in most	Arthritis in 2% who get shigella, salmonella, yersinia, campylobacter or *C. difficile* overall but in 20% of infected who are HLA B27+
Crohn's disease	Arhritis 20%. AS 10%. Sacroiliitis in 26%	60% of spondylarthropathy patients have histological evidence of bowel nflammation. See also below
Ulcerative colitis	Arthritis 20%. AS 7%. Sacroiliitis 15%	See also above. Severity of gut and joint inflammation varies in its association but SIJ/spine inflammation does not
Whipple's disease	Migratory arthritis in >60%	*T. whippelii* identified in small bowel. Diarrhoea occurs in >75% ultimately
Intestinal by-pass surgery (blind loop syndrome)	Polyarticular symptoms 50% in scleroderma	Intestinal bacterial overgrowth in small bowel. ?Associated with joint symptoms
Coeliac disease	Arthritis is rare	?Increased intestinal permeability
Viral enteritis	Rare (<0.5%)	Most common: coxsackie or echo
Hepatitis A	Arthralgia 15%. Vasculitis rare	Causal association
Hepatitis B	Arthralgia 10–25%. PAN	Aetiological. Vasculitis in 50% HBsAg carriers
Hepatitis C	Sialadenitis in >50%. Vasculitis (cryoglobulinaemic)	?Aetiological in Sjögren's. Hepatitis C identified in 27–96% of patients with cryoglobulinaemia
Primary biliary cirrhosis	Polyarthritis 19%. Scleroderma 18%. Sjögren's 50%	Autoimmune 'overlap'. Features may be subclinical
Chronic active hepatitis	Polyarthralgia or arthritis in 25–50%	Autoimmunity
Hemochromatosis	OA 50%	Iron storage disease
Wilson's disease	OA in 50% adults. Chondrocalcinosis	Copper storage disease

Table 4.7 Gut and hepatobiliary manifestations in rheumatological diseases (I: General)

Disease	Abnormalities	Presentation with
Rheumatoid arthritis	TMJ arthritis Oesophageal dysmotility	Impaired mastication Dysphagia, reflux
	GI vasculitis (0.1%)	Ulcers, pain, infarction
	Portal hypertension	Splenomegaly (Felty's)
	Liver involvement (Felty's)	Enzyme abnormalities
	Hepatosplenomegaly	Palpable viscera
Systemic lupus erythematosus	Oesophageal dysmotility	Dysphagia, reflux
	GI vasculitis	Ulcers, pain, perforation
	Protein-losing enteropathy	Hypoalbuminaemia
	Peritonitis	Ascites (10%), serositis
	Hepatosplenomegaly (30%)	Palpable viscera
Scleroderma	Oesophageal dysmotility	Heartburn/dysphagia
	Delayed gastric emptying	Aggravated reflux
	Intestinal dysmotility and fibrosis (80%)	Malabsorption, pseudo-obstruction (<1%)
	Pseudo and wide mouth diverticulae	Haemorrhage, stasis, bacterial overgrowth
Polymyositis and dermatomyositis	Muscle weakness	Aspiration, dysphagia
	Disordered motility	Dysphagia, constipation
	Vasculitis (rare)	Ulcers, perforation
MCTD	Hypomotility	Dysphagia, reflux, pseudo-obstruction
Sjögren's syndrome	Membrane dessication	Xerostomia, dysphagia
	Oesophageal webs (10%)	Dysphagia (>60%)
	Gastric infiltrates/atrophy	Masses, dyspepsia
	Pancreatitis	Pain, amylasaemia
	Hepatic dysfunction	Hepatomegaly (≅25%)
	Hepatic cirrhosis	Primary biliary cirrhosis
Spondylarthritis	Ileocolonic inflammation	May be asymptomatic
Adult onset Still's	Hepatitis, peritonitis, hepatosplenomegaly	Pain or abnormal enzymes (≅75%)
Systemic JIA	Serositis	Abdominal pain
	Hepatomegaly	Abnormal enzymes
Marfan, Ehlers-Danlos	Defective collagen	Hypomotility, Malabsorption, visceral rupture/laxity

- Gut amyloid is present in 21% of RA patients (autopsy study). In some, (non-gut) amyloid was considered the cause of death.
- The rate of deaths from amyloid in JIA has ↓ from 42 to 17% since the 1970s due to aggressive treatment.
- Amyloid can be diagnosed from rectal (75% diagnostic yield), lip (86% yield) or subcutaneous fat biopsy. Characteristic patterns of deposition are recognized with ^{111}In-labelled serum amyloid-P scintigraphy.
- Quite severe GI disturbances can coexist with relatively stable limited cutaneous scleroderma, i.e. skin and gut disease does not necessarily correlate. Overall GI problems are extremely frequent.
- In SLE serious gut and hepatobiliary manifestations are relatively uncommon (5%) though nausea, anorexia, vomiting, and diarrhoea are quite frequent.
- GI vasculitis is associated with virtually all the autoimmune connective tissue diseases and is part of systemic vasculitides (see Table 4.8). It can present in a variety of ways such as with non-specific features such as abdominal pain, anorexia, and anaemia or with an 'acute abdomen' in patients with established disease. It can also be the disease-presenting feature.

Gut and hepatobiliary side-effects from drugs used in treating rheumatological and bone diseases

Such side-effects are common:

- NSAIDs should be considered as potentially toxic as some other drugs used for rheumatological diseases including immunosuppressive drugs.
- Peptic ulcers and gastroduodenal erosions appear to occur less frequently with selective cyclo-oxygenase II (COX II)-inhibiting NSAIDs such as celecoxib, etoricoxib, valdecoxib and meloxicam than with NSAIDs that inhibit COX II less selectively.
- Glucocorticoids are (rarely) associated with peptic ulceration, perforation and pancreatitis. The latter two are unusual at doses <12.5 mg/day.
- Methotrexate gut and hepatobiliary side effects are relatively common. Abdominal pain, nausea, vomiting, diarrhoea, stomati-tis/mouth, ulcers and altered taste occur. All may respond to dose reduction. Liver enzyme elevation occurs in up to 88% at some time during treatment. Serious hepatic disease is unusual, though cirrhosis is a risk. Children typically tolerate higher doses than adults (even up to 10–50 mg/week).
- IM gold can cause mouth ulcers (5–20%). Diarrhoea is rare (1%) with IM but common with oral gold (40%). Significant liver disease and enterocolitis occur with both forms but are rare.

Table 4.8 Gut and hepatobiliary manifestations in rheumatological diseases (II Vasculitis)

Disease	Frequency of GI vasculitis and features
Polyarteritis nodosa	80% (mesenteric). Buccal ulcers, cholecystitis (15%), bowel infarction, perforation, appendicitis, pancreatitis, strictures, chronic wasting syndrome
Henoch–Schönlein Purpura	44–68%. Abdominal pain, meleana, haematemesis, ulcers, intussusception, cholecystitis, infarction, perforation, appendicitis
Churg–Strauss Syndrome	≅40%. Haemorrhage, ulceration, infarction, perforation
Behçet's syndrome	Buccal and intestinal ulcers, haemorrhage, perforation, pyloric stenosis, rectal ulcers
Systemic lupus erythematosus	2%. Buccal ulcers, ileocolitis, gastritis, ulceration, perforation, intussusception, volvulus (1%), pneumatosis
Kawasaki disease	Abdominal pain, intestinal obstruction, non-infective diarrhoea
Wegener's granulomatosis	<5%. Cholecystitis, appendicitis, ileocolitis, infarction
Juvenile dermatomyositis	Well recognized. Perforation, pneumatosis
MCTD	Rare. Ulceration, perforation, pancreatitis
RA (including RF+ JIA)	0.1%. Buccal ulcers, abdominal pain, peptic ulcers, acalculus cholecystitis, gut infarction, and perforation
Polymyositis and dermatomyositis	Very rare. Mucosal ulcers, perforation and pneumatosis
Cryoglobulinaemia	Rare. Ischaemia and infarction

- Sulphasalazine gut and hepatobiliary side-effects are common and may occur in up to 20% of patients. The most frequent are mostly mild: indigestion, nausea, vomiting, anorexia, and abdominal pain. Gut ulceration, bloody diarrhoea, and serious liver problems are rare. In about 65% of side-effects occur in the first 3 months of treatment.
- Azathioprine can cause nausea (15%), vomiting (10%), and abdominal pain (8%). Diarrhoea is rare (5%). Liver enzyme abnormalities are often mild and may remit on lowering the dose. The GI side effects are not always dependent on TPMT status.
- D-penicillamine causes altered taste (25% within the first 3–6 months), nausea or vomiting (18%), and stomatitis/mouth ulcers (5%). Hepatotoxicity and haemorrhagic colitis are rare.

- Chloroquine and hydroxychloroquine, used in mild SLE particularly, can cause non-specific GI intolerance (10%). The onset is often insidious.
- Ciclosporin causes gingival hyperplasia, nausea, diarrhoea, and elevation in hepatic enzymes.
- Effects of cyclophosphamide on the gut are frequent and include nausea, vomiting, diarrhoea, and stomatitis. Serious hepatotoxicity is rare.
- Chlorambucil has a low incidence of GI side-effects.
- Leflunomide can cause nausea (8–13%), diarrhoea (up to 25%), and abnormal liver enzymes. In studies to date, most rises in transaminases have been mild (< two-fold) and are reversible on drug withdrawal.
- Oral bisphosphonates, given for osteoporosis, such as alendronate and risedronate can cause nausea, dyspepsia, and diarrhoea. Oesophageal ulceration has occasionally been noted with alendronate though it is thought this occurs only in people who do not follow the instructions for taking them. Myoarthralgias can also occur.
- Strontium ranelate is as well-tolerated as placebo in all studies but can cause GI side-effects. Extensive post-marketing data on side-effects are not yet available.
- Calcitonin either given as s/c injection or as nasal spray can give abdominal pains and diarrhoea.

Malignancy

Rheumatic features may be clues to the existence of cancer and may be caused either by direct invasion or indirectly as a paraneoplastic syndrome.

Primary and secondary neoplastic diseases of bone and joints

- Synovial tumours are rare. Sarcoma (synovioma) is commoner in men than women and unusual in those over 60. It usually occurs in the legs (70%) and can occur around tendon sheaths and bursae. At diagnosis, pulmonary metastases are common.
- Para-articular involvement by bone tumours may give a monoarticular effusion. Invasion of synovium may occur and malignant cells can be detected in joint fluid. Breast, bronchogenic carcinoma, GI tumours, and melanoma can all metastasize to joints.
- Lymphomas and leukaemias may simulate various conditions and cause synovitis in a single or in multiple joints.
- Arthritis complicating presentation of myeloma or an acute leukaemia is most likely to be polyarticular asymmetrical.
- In adults, arthritis complicating leukaemia is rare (5% of cases).
- Leukaemia is the most frequent malignancy in Caucasian children and the most frequent cause of neoplastic skeletal symptoms in childhood and adolescence (15% of leukaemia cases).
- Neuroblastomas are the most frequent cause of a solid tumour metastasizing to the skeleton in children.

Clues that may lead to a suspicion of malignancy directly causing musculoskeletal symptoms

- Constitutional symptoms.
- Migratory arthralgia/arthritis.
- The coexistence of bone pain (also consider metabolic bone diseases, sarcoid, and enthesitis-related conditions).
- Haemorrhagic joint fluid (also consider trauma, pigmented villonodular synovitis (PVNS), chondrocalcinosis).
- Radiographs that show adjacent bone destruction, perhaps with loss of cortex (also consider infection).
- Radiographic calcification in soft-tissue mass (?synovioma).

Paraneoplastic myopathies

Paraneoplastic myopathies may occur at the time of presentation of malignancy, precede it sometimes by months to years, follow its treatment, or occur as a complication of established disease:

- Myopathy is usually due to carcinomatous neuromyopathy. Poly/dermatomyositis, Eaton–Lambert myasthenic syndrome (ELMS) and hypophosphataemic (oncogenic) osteomalacia are associated with, though not specific for, malignancy (see Table 4.9).
- Carcinomatous neuromyopathy is a condition characterized by symmetrical muscle weakness and wasting. The myopathy can pre-date malignancy.

Table 4.9 Myopathy and links with malignancy

Condition	Typical pattern of weakness	Common cancer associations	Other features
Carcinomatous neuromyopathy	Pelvic girdle—symmetrical	Lung: 15% men, 12% women. Ovary: 16%. Stomach: 7% men, 13% women	Wasting, EMG abnormality, and increase in muscle enzymes are not invariable
Dermatomyositis (+?PM)	Proximal limb. Truncal	Reflects underlying cancer frequency in local population	Response to steroids is usual
Myasthenia gravis (MG)	Frequently ocular and bulbar muscles involved	Thymus. Any	Muscle strength fluctuates (fatiguability). Responds to anti-cholinesterases
Eaton–Lambert myasthenic syndrome (ELMS)	Pelvic girdle muscles. Altered gait. Ocular muscles not affected	Small cell lung. Can occur up to 2–3 years after ELMS	Autonomic disturbances. EMG + poor response to anticholinesterase distinguish from MG
Oncogenic osteomalacia	Generalized. Develops insidiously	Small discrete mesenchymal tumours in bone, soft tissues, and sinuses. Neurofibromatosis	Bone pain and bone demineralization. Hypophosphataemia and low circulating 1,25 vitamin D

Investigations

The following investigations are recommended for patients presenting with a form of cancer-related myopathy:

- To confirm muscle disease consider: FBC/CBC; measures of acute phase; muscle enzymes; EMG; muscle biopsy; autoantibodies, e.g. ANA, anti-RNP and anti-Jo1 (PM) and anti-acetylcholine receptor antibodies in MG.
- Rapid relief of symptoms with IV injection of edrophonium (up to 10 mg) is typical in MG but unlikely in ELMS. Prior injection of atropine 0.2 mg protects against antimuscarinic effects.
- A search for malignancy is essential. Suspicious clinical features will guide the focus and extent of the search. Frequent associations are shown in Table 4.9.
- Imaging studies need to be thorough and include skeletal scintigraphy and usually thoracoabdominal cavity studies.
- Other investigations to consider: chest radiograph and skeletal survey, ovarian and bowel tumour markers, mammography, PSA, serum protein electrophoresis.
- Surveillance for the appearance of tumours if initial investigations are unrevealing is prudent. Tumour appearance may be a few years after the onset of myopathy in some cases.

Non-myopathic paraneoplastic syndromes

The non-myopathic paraneoplastic syndromes are rare:

- Hypertrophic osteoarthropathy (HO) consists of clubbing, periostitis of tubular bones, and an arthropathy (may range from arthralgia to diffuse polyarthritis). Suspicion of this should prompt a request for an isotope bone scan which typically shows abnormally ↑ bone turnover in the long bones. Radiographs often show periosteal elevation.
- HO complicates 20% of primary lung tumours (thus 'hypertrophic *pulmonary* osteoarthropathy') though it is associated with other malignancies.
- Polyarthritis may be the presenting feature of cancer. Most cases occur in those aged over 60. Nodules and deformities do not occur as in RA and it is less likely to be symmetrical though both occur in multicentric reticulohistiocytosis—which is malignancy-asso-ciated and might be mistaken for RA.
- Eosinophilic fasciitis, severe bilateral palmar fasciitis (often mistaken for scleroderma), and fasciitis associated with panniculitis have been associated with malignancy. Cases of 'shoulder–hand' syndrome with cancer probably reflect similar pathological processes.

Rheumatic diseases associated with an increased incidence of malignancy

There are a number of rheumatic diseases that are associated with an increased incidence of malignancy compared with healthy populations. Data gathering in this area has been difficult. Only the strongest data are reflected here.

- The most highly associated cancer in RA is non-Hodgkin's lymphoma. Paraproteinaemia and myeloma are also associated.
- RA patients may be partially protected from colorectal cancer owing to the chronic effects of NSAIDs on bowel mucosa.
- Use of cyclophosphamide and chlorambucil is associated with an ↑ cancer risk but use of methotrexate and azathioprine is probably not.
- Non-Hodgkin's B-cell lymphoma develops in a subset of patients with Sjögren's syndrome (4%). Its onset may be indicated by rapid enlargement of salivary glands, the appearance of a paraprotein, or decrease in circulating immunoglobulins or RF titre.
- The association between malignancy and SLE or scleroderma is controversial. Cases may relate to use of cyclophosphamide.
- DM is probably associated with malignancy in adults, though convincing evidence for an association of PM with malignancy is lacking. Neither is associated with malignancy in children.
- There are no specific clinical or laboratory features which discriminate DM associated with malignancy from the 'uncomplicated' disease, although weight loss and a negative ANA should raise the possibility of a malignancy-related condition. Close surveillance for a tumour in the first year after DM (+?PM) diagnosis in those >45 years of age is justified.

Index

T

U

V

W